Advance praise for Thinking Themselves FREE

"*Thinking Themselves Free: Research on the Literacy of Teen Mothers* is a powerful multilayered Narrative of the stories of teen mothers, teachers of teen mothers, and the life of one researcher as she struggles to understand the lives of the teens and to uncover the intricate web of fictions that surround teen motherhood. Cynthia Miller Coffel not only interviews young mothers, she shares her own journey as a teacher and researcher working with teen moms' programs. As you read *Thinking Themselves Free,* you may find, as I did, some troubling stereotypes that you carry within because of the available fictions of females that remain so pervasive in our culture. In telling the stories of teen mothers, Miller Coffel introduces readers to complex people living complex lives. Throughout this book, Miller Coffel is compassionate, yet never sentimental. This is a beautifully written narrative that complicates what it means to be poor and pregnant, to want to be a 'helper of the poor,' and importantly, about literacy teaching and learning and how schools might work."

—*Margaret J. Finders, Professor of English, University of Wisconsin La Crosse;*
Author of Just Girls: Hidden Literacies and Life in Junior High

Thinking Themselves
FREE

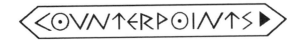

Studies in the Postmodern Theory of Education

Shirley R. Steinberg
General Editor

Vol. 389

The Counterpoints series is part of the Peter Lang Education list.
Every volume is peer reviewed and meets
the highest quality standards for content and production.

PETER LANG
New York • Washington, D.C./Baltimore • Bern
Frankfurt • Berlin • Brussels • Vienna • Oxford

Cynthia Miller Coffel

Thinking Themselves
FREE

Research on the Literacy of Teen Mothers

Montante Family Library
D'Youville College

PETER LANG
New York • Washington, D.C./Baltimore • Bern
Frankfurt • Berlin • Brussels • Vienna • Oxford

Library of Congress Cataloging-in-Publication Data
Miller Coffel, Cynthia.
Thinking themselves free: research on the literacy of teen mothers /
Cynthia Miller Coffel.
p. cm. – (Counterpoints: studies in the postmodern theory
of education; v. 389)
Includes bibliographical references and index.
1. Teenage mothers. 2. Teenage pregnancy. I. Title.
HQ759.4.M554   306.874'3–dc22   2010014267
ISBN 978-1-4331-0973-7 (hardcover)
ISBN 978-1-4331-0972-0 (paperback)
ISSN 1058-1634

Bibliographic information published by **Die Deutsche Nationalbibliothek**.
Die Deutsche Nationalbibliothek lists this publication in the "Deutsche
Nationalbibliografie"; detailed bibliographic data is available
on the Internet at http://dnb.d-nb.de/.

FSC
Mixed Sources
Product group from well-managed
forests, controlled sources and
recycled wood or fiber

Cert no. SCS-COC-002464
www.fsc.org
©1996 Forest Stewardship Council

Cover design by Kate Jones

The paper in this book meets the guidelines for permanence and durability
of the Committee on Production Guidelines for Book Longevity
of the Council of Library Resources.

Table of Contents

Acknowledgments

Thanks are due to my advisers at the University of Iowa: Cynthia Lewis, Anne DiPardo, Gail Boldt, Carolyn Colvin, Mary Trachsel, and James Marshall, who taught me how to conduct qualitative research and provided me with intellectual sustenance as I wrestled with the new and old ideas that inform this work. As I worked on revisions, I was fortunate to have the help of five good readers: Scott Coffel, Marilyn Fehn, Andrew H. Miller, Nina Metzner, and Jim Patterson, each of whom, pen in hand, reviewed part or all of this work as it progressed from a dissertation to a series of articles to an almost-finished draft. I am grateful as well for the kindness of Mary Stein and Cindy Erenberger, who opened up time in my workday so I could conduct this research.

I greatly appreciated the help of Shirley Steinberg, Chris Meyers, and Sophie Appel from Peter Lang Publishing, who chose to include this book in their series and guided me through production; but it wouldn't have been a book without the work of Kate Jones, graphic artist extraordinaire. Thanks especially to the early morning coffee girls and the google group gym girls—you know who you are—for sustaining me with encouragement, insight and laughter at the top of the stairs most weekdays.

Five young mothers were brave to open up to me: Without their willingness to tell the true stories of their lives there would be no book. Teachers and counselors took time to answer my questions and pose their own: Young women's lives are a little less harsh because the people whose wisdom I describe in these pages are still at work.

My deepest gratitude is to my family: Lou Horton and William Lee Miller, Rebecca Uchida, David Miller, and Andrew H. Miller, who talked to me about this book in Bloomington, Chicago, New York, and Virginia, in e-mails, phone calls, at Christmas celebrations and at a couple of 80th-birthday parties.

This book was written in the company of Scott and Ethan Coffel. It is my life with them that matters most.

Permissions

Portions of Chapter 3 appeared in the *International Journal of Qualitative Studies in Education*, volume 15, no 6. Copyright Routledge (2009). Reprinted with permission from the *International Journal of Qualitative Studies in Education*.

Portions of Chapter 5 appeared in *The ALAN Review*, volume 35, no 3. Copyright by the National Council of Teachers of English (2008). Used with permission.

Portions of Interludes 2, 3, and 4 appeared in *WILLA: A Journal of the Women in Literature and Life Assembly of the National Council of Teachers of English*, volume 8. Copyright by the National Council of Teachers of English (1999). Used with permission.

Chapter 1

Marginal and Secret Stories

This . . . is about lives lived out on the borderlands, lives for which the central interpretive devices of the culture don't quite work.

—Carolyn Steedman, 1986

Thirty years ago, when I was just twenty-four, I taught English for a year at the Teen Moms' Program, a school for married, pregnant, and mothering teens in a small city in Utah. Back then the old brick Johnson High School building on 20th Street housed all of the students who didn't belong in the regular high schools: gifted students, who wanted to study higher mathematics or practice chess; refugees from Laos, Cambodia, and Vietnam; young men who had done jail time for stealing cars or dealing drugs; and the women I was supposed to teach, the young mothers.

I suppose anyone's first teaching job is strange. It's uncomfortable to be thrust into a position of authority before you really feel ready, even though you've spent so many years reading all those books—*What Do I Do Monday?* and *Up the Down Staircase* and *Don't Smile Until Christmas*—that are supposed to tell you what teaching is like, but never can. I know I was scared, walking up the cement steps and through the double doors, past the principal's office, by the rooms that the gifted kids had named the Youth Eager for Truth School and the ESL center where wrinkled old refugees in their bright strange clothing learned how to pronounce their vowels. When I climbed the stairs to the second floor and the Teen Moms' Program, boys from the school for kids just out of jail stood around the stairwell, following my ascent and whistling under their breath, sometimes howling.

In my classroom—a room that always seemed too big to me, with a blue rug, a baby-bottle warmer, a leftover mobile dangling over my desk, and completely empty bookshelves—on that first day, I was suddenly staring at six girls sitting around tables. This was my child development class; it was an hour and a half long; I planned to cover the first six weeks of life that day. Even though I'd participated in the school's registration week, finding students' information in a big book at my table, talking with their mothers, or being introduced to their babies in strollers; even though, during that week, I'd heard about the girl who'd borrowed a neighbor's baby so she could prove that she was a mother and enroll; even though I'd been told stories about how angry boyfriends sometimes showed up at the school and had to be dragged away by the police; even though I'd seen the daycare center across the hall and fixed up my bulletin board with cutouts of Raggedy Ann and Andy, seeing real students, with their diaper bags and their notebooks, sitting at tables in front of me was something of a shock. These girls didn't look the way "pregnant teenagers" or "teen mothers," whom I was there to help, had looked in my imagination. They all seemed to be holding babies in their arms. They were all more knowledgeable about the subject of baby-raising, of child development, than I was, I realized. I wanted to run out the door.

One girl smiled helpfully and then calmly lifted up her shirt, pulled out a breast, and began nursing her daughter. Another came in late, glancing at me defiantly, I thought, pulling her son in a little red wagon behind her. I tried to introduce myself to the girls and ignore them at the same time; I tried to shut them out of my vision and greet them warmly, too. I sat behind my desk and began reading aloud from my notes about the first few hours of life, about what babies really look like when they're born, and about the importance of letting the dried-up remnants of the umbilical cord fall off the baby's belly by itself. One girl interrupted me mid-sentence. "I hear my baby crying," she said, and before I could stop her, she stood up and walked out of the room.

"I'm gonna puke," said another girl, who ran out the door, holding her stomach.

The nursing girl's braces glittered when she smiled. She looked at me appraisingly as her tiny baby suckled. "You're a first-year teacher, aren't you," she said.

I learned a lot that year: among other things, about how Brigham Young came to marry fifty-five women, how to ski cross-country, how Rudolph Dreikurs recommends that parents use "natural consequences" in disciplining their children, how to say "queer" in Thai, how to burp a baby, how to get into the Celestial, or highest, of the three Mormon heavens, how to make Nigerian stew, how dead bodies are embalmed, and what's so important, to the people of Utah, about the Golden Spike.

It was a combination of a yearning for adventure, a liberal religious conviction that all of us deserve a second chance, and a feminist concern for women—I'd studied feminism and modernism with Gilbert and Gubar the year before I went out to Utah—that took me to the Teen Moms' Program. It was stubbornness and a refusal to quit despite all my many mistakes that kept me there a whole year.

Partly, I went to Utah to teach in a school for unwed mothers with the thought, there but for the grace of God, go I. It could be me, surely, I thought, a teenager with a child and no husband. Hadn't I, once or twice, said yes when I'd wanted to say no? Hadn't I, once or twice, prayed for my period to appear? But the girls I taught were different from me in many ways, I discovered; I discovered that my empathy for them, or rather, my identification with them, was wrongheaded in some ways, and in some ways naive. I was different from the young women I taught not simply in age—they were adolescents in a time very different from the time in which I had been an adolescent—and not simply in that we grew up in different parts of the country, with different discourses predominating—the Mormon belief that the best thing a woman can do in life is to have children surely influenced many of my students—but I was different from those young women in that I was affluent, and came from a successful home, and most of my students were not affluent, and did not come from successful homes. Kristin Luker (1996), author of *Dubious Conceptions: The Politics of Teenage Pregnancy*, writes that "typically, a young person ends up as a teenage parent only after going through a series of steps, and at each step the successful and affluent are screened out" (114). She writes that although middle-class young women do become pregnant out of wedlock, those women are more likely to have abortions than poorer girls are:

> About 40 percent of pregnant teens seek an abortion; those who seek abortions tend to be affluent and white, to have more ambitious educational and career goals, and to have higher grade point averages. All these factors taken together mean that affluent teens, a bit more than 60 percent of the age group, account for fewer than a fifth of all early births. Furthermore, middle-class and affluent teens who do get pregnant and who do not seek an abortion are much more likely to marry than poor ones. (115)

Luker goes on to say that those poorer women who do have children young "are often the more discouraged of the disadvantaged" (115). These are generalizations, of course, and in these pages we will meet both poor young mothers who are not discouraged and working-and middle-class women who have chosen to give birth to children conceived out of wedlock. Still, the majority of the girls who came to the Teen Moms' Program were poor, and in that I was not, and not often discouraged, I was wrong to believe that I would see much of myself in the young women I taught at the Teen Moms'

Program.

But I came to feel as if I were an older sister to some of those girls. When one group started a man-hating club, I felt sorry that they were so bitter so young, and yet I shared some of their anger—not to say rage—at the opposite sex who seem to have it so easy in our society. I shared some of the shyness, the dependent behaviors of my students, as well as some of the confusion about sexuality, and about power negotiations with members of the opposite sex. At the same time I often felt out of touch as I tried to teach English and child development and health and foods and children's literature and creative writing and economics and comparative religions: a religion professor's daughter, I was surprised to learn that the student in high heels really was a prostitute; a feminist decidedly uninterested in the domestic, I had trouble getting excited when a student told me she'd bought a new washing machine; a lover of literature, an always-intent reader, I had trouble understanding girls whose favorite reading material was *Cosmo*.

I struggled to learn how to teach that year and despite what I've heard about how education courses don't help teachers once they're out in the real world, that year I used every single thing I had learned in my methods class. In my English class students read literature I'd chosen in graduate school, in a series of lesson plans centered on the life stories of women of courage who had babies out of wedlock. I had students read and talk, in those lessons, about the last chapter of *I Know Why the Caged Bird Sings*, in which Maya Angelou describes the birth of her son, when she was nineteen; I had students read angry newspaper articles about Ingrid Bergman's bastard child, a funny essay from Nikki Giovanni's memoir *Gemini*, called, "Don't Have a Baby Until You Read This," and an essay by the Catholic reformer Dorothy Day about the birth of her daughter out of wedlock. Following other plans I'd made in my education courses, I taught a mini course on death in literature, in which we wrote our own obituaries, acted out a portion of *Our Town*, and walked down the street for a tour of the local mortuary. I took students to a Buddhist temple in town and had a social worker come in and talk about depression.

One of the best ideas I had in that English class was to go out and buy, at a secondhand bookstore, every young-adult novel I could find that had anything to do with teenage pregnancy. I handed out those books, asking that my students write two-page reports on the ones they chose. I don't think anyone turned in their book reports but I know those novels were read with intensity. Months later I'd hear girls telling each other the plot of *Don't Look and It Won't Hurt*, or referring to *Mr. and Mrs. Bo Jo Jones* in class. Girls who were not in my classes came to me asking for more books about "girls like us." A book called *I Want to Keep My Baby!*, which later became a made-for-TV movie, was particularly popular. I never got my copy of that novel back.

I wondered then, how did the stories my students read match up with the stories they were living? Bits of those girls' lives stay with me persistently: Star, who tried so hard to figure out how to discipline her beloved daughter, Heaven, and felt such remorse after hitting her with a hairbrush; Sylvia, who wanted to become a psychologist, and whose ranch-owning grandmother wouldn't let her ride her favorite Appaloosa after she became pregnant; Amie, whose water broke at a rock concert; Carmen, who said, "I'm bad, yeah! My teacher called me a dirty Mexican and I pushed him down the stairs!"; Heather, who said she resented her daughter 80% of the time, and whose parents were trying to arrest her boyfriend for statutory rape; Toya, who worked two jobs while trying to finish high school so she could live on her own with her daughter and they could "be a family"; Erin, whose mother had her arrested for abusing her baby son; Laurie, who ran away to Arizona with her son, a diaper bag, and all the money the school had collected for a Thanksgiving dance; Rosie Jaramillo, an eighteen-year-old mother of two who gave a defense so sharp at the Utah High School-Teen Moms' Program mock trial that our consulting lawyer shook his head and said he wished she could go to law school; and Carla Ortega, a fourteen-year-old and a talented writer whose boyfriend started out as her baby sitter. Surely the stories in the young-adult literature those students read were nowhere near as complicated as the stories of those students' lives.

So how did the girls think about those books? How would they have told their own stories to me, if I had formally asked them? How did the discourses around those girls, in the novels I gave them and elsewhere, affect the ways they thought about themselves? I wonder how those girls fit their experiences into the larger stories that society tells about women, about teenage girls, and about teen mothers in particular. I wonder how their lives and identities were shaped by the institutions they lived in and around—school and family—and by the ways people in those institutions thought about literacy.

Reading about women, autobiography, and narrative now, I learn that even women of accomplishment have a hard time telling true stories of their lives, because most biographies and autobiographies written and told throughout history have been the stories of men, and men's life stories create templates, or master stories, into which women's lives don't quite fit. And when women's life stories have been told, throughout history they have been told most often by men, and described as following the arc that men decide upon, emphasizing, perhaps, romance over accomplishment, passivity over persistence, and luck over striving. I learn that some of the stories I had my students read the year that I taught at the Teen Moms' Program, those autobiographies of courageous women, were, in this way, not really honest: Dorothy Day is one of many who, Carolyn Heilbrun (1988) suggests, made the story of her life far simpler and far more conventionally feminine than it really was. Like many female autobiographers, Day told stories "written in the old genre of female autobiography, which tends to find beauty even in pain and to transform rage into spiritual acceptance" (12). In telling her own story, Day did not "protest against the available fiction of female becoming" (18).

The young-adult novels that I had my students read were also influenced by the prevailing fictions about women's lives. The identities those novels presented to my students were rather conventional ones. Which of those plots would my students borrow and revise to tell their own life stories? The young mothers' life stories were, in some ways, typical female stories, with childbirth, not work, at their centers; and yet in other ways the young mothers' stories were not typical, since by having babies in adolescence, these women do not follow the accepted middle-class female "relation between chronology and plot" (Lesko 1998, 125). These young mothers were certainly not feminists, and yet they were struggling within and against discourses that have structured many women's lives. They were struggling with issues that most women in our society must think about, issues of economics, dependency, equality, care, assertion, commitment, and the relationship of the self to the body.

Learning how in-school and out-of-school literacies, and experiences in school, had shaped the lives of a small group of young mothers might help teachers, teacher educators, and school administrators think in new ways about the education of teen mothers. Such a study might help school administrators see how the education of teen mothers is an equity issue in the schools; it might help teacher educators think about new ways of preparing teachers to work with this clientele; it might help educate some teachers about the literate lives of the teen mothers in their classrooms. The lives of teen mothers have primarily been studied by psychologists and sociologists, not by educators, and not in relation to school. How would my students have answered if I had asked them to tell me how schooling experiences and experiences with reading and writing had influenced the direction of their lives?

I wanted to ask some of the questions I've listed above to the young mothers I had known so long ago. Married now, mother of a son, entrenched in my own middle-aged, middle-class life, I couldn't go back and talk with those girls. So, as is my habit, twenty-five years after that first year of teaching, I began to read.

Available Fictions

In his little book *Making Stories: Law, Literature, and Life*, the great philosopher of education Jerome Bruner (2003) writes that stories reside somewhere in the tension between supporting the conventional and subverting or transgressing it. He writes that great stories are in some ways deeply and always about "plight" (20), about the difficulty of being human. Bruner describes stories, particularly autobiographical ones, as "acts of mind" (76), of which there may be many versions, and many of which are "advertisements for a right selfhood, each with its own version of the tempting competition" (77). I believe that the young women with whom I speak in this book work hard to provide advertisements for a right selfhood; their stories are certainly about the difficulty of being human.

In the chapters that follow I'll explore the question of how these young women, through reading and writing, through taking bits of the discourses around them and rejecting others, try to construct new and more generative life stories for themselves. Which parts of these discourses do they accept and which do they reject? Inside that large question are smaller ones, particular to the experiences I had with these young women, like, what are their literacy histories and how have those affected their lives and identities? How do they react to the discourses we discover in the young-adult novels we read and how does their autobiographical writing interact with those discourses? How do the stories they read and write match up with the stories they've lived?

Those discourses that affect the way the young women in this book tell their stories affect the ways public policy about teen mothers is shaped as well. Deirdre Kelly (2000), in *Pregnant with Meaning: Teen Mothers and the Politics of Inclusive Schooling*, and Wendy Luttrell (2003), in *Pregnant Bodies, Fertile Minds: Gender, Race, and the Schooling of Pregnant Teens*, describe four groups who express competing discourses about teen mothers. As each group looks at teen mothers and pregnant teenagers, they see different reasons for the young women's out-of-wedlock pregnancies, and different solutions to the "problem" of teenage mothering.

Some people concerned with the lives of teen mothers speak through what Kelly (2000) calls a "wrong-girl" frame (74). This way of thinking suggests that there is something wrong with the girl, that she is rebellious or confused, without goals, overly sexual, or irresponsible in the way she thinks about relationships, parenting, boys, or her body. This is the dominant way of thinking around teenage pregnancy and motherhood; according to Kelly, it holds the most power of the four discourses listed here. Perhaps it is the most powerful because it's connected to the language that, according to studies conducted by Nancy Lesko (1996), sees youth itself as a "major social problem," comprised of young people who fail to follow "proper norms for development and are prone to violence, pregnancy, motherhood, school dropout, unemployment, and other deviances" (as cited in Boler 1999, 89). This "wrong-girl" discourse is difficult to unravel not only because it holds some truth, as all of these four ways of thinking do, but because it includes a discourse of "people who make bad choices" (Kelly 2000, 47) that attempts to separate the deed from the doer in a way that seems well motivated. But this way of thinking is unfortunate because it overlooks the difficulties created by poverty—the ways in which young women in particular are called upon to do the emotional and practical work of keeping troubled families together (Dodson 1998) and the isolation this causes; as well as the lure and danger of relationships with young men, who are themselves often under brutal economic pressures. This way of thinking about teenage motherhood is an example of the insidiousness of the ideology of individualism and of the lack of complexity of our understanding of how poverty affects psychology. In addition, this way of thinking about teenage parenting is unfortunate because it does not take into account the many and conflicting messages young women receive about sexuality today; it does not take into account the ways young women and girls are "eroticized" in everyday life (Luttrell 2003, 33).

The "wrong-society" frame is one first expressed by feminists; this frame concerns itself not only with young women's lack of access to birth control but also with a struggle over "proper family-government relationships" (Luttrell 2003, 35). Arguing that individual choices should be seen in context of the society in which those choices are made, those who see teen mothers through this frame suggest that our society, in which men's health comes first, should change to address the needs of young women, and the poor in general, more aggressively.

Those who speak through a "wrong-family frame" say that the family is at fault: the family of the pregnant teenager has raised their daughter badly. This construction dates back to the 1960s and the Moynihan Report which spoke of the problems of the black family; this construction also connects to the culture of poverty discourse that describes undeserving mothers who are on welfare and criminal, absent fathers. As Nancy Lesko (1995) put it, this framework has been used as "part of a broad social engineering toward reprivatization and dismantlement of the welfare state support of women and children" (as quoted in Luttrell 2003, 34).

Finally, there are some teen mothers who claim that any stigma about having children out of wedlock is wrong. Kelly (2000) and others (Edin & Kefelas 2005; Luttrell 2003; Lycke 2010; Schultz 2001) have described teen mothers' self-interpretations as emphasizing the positive and empowering aspects of their situations. Schultz describes the ways three girls she got to know at an urban high school turned "failure into success" as they struggled with ideas about teenage mothering, ideas that affected the ways they saw themselves as well as the way society saw them. Schultz suggests that—as with the young women I spoke to—"a consequence of having children at a young age can lead to new forms of participation in school" (595).

Though public images of the teen mother fluctuate, in recent times the prevalent image of the black pregnant teenager and teen mother has become a focal point where societal anxieties about female power and about poverty, about sex and youth and race have coalesced (Luker 1996). We have been fascinated by the teen mother and intent on demonizing her for some time now, even though, as Luker writes, women who become pregnant out of wedlock are more likely to be in their early twenties than to be teenagers. And although teen mothers are often constructed as the cause of poverty and welfare dependency, reducing rates of teenage pregnancy, and reducing out-of-wedlock pregnancy, would not make a significant dent in government welfare spending (Kelly 2000; Luker 1996); it's an open question whether becoming pregnant young and out of wedlock disrupts poor girls' already-lousy life opportunities (Edin & Kefelas 2005, 48).

The question of how schools should work with teen mothers and pregnant teens is an open one, too. Luker (1996) writes of the "cultural schizophrenia" exhibited in our society around the issue of young parenting and teenage pregnancy. She explains that while we expect women to "emulate competitive, selfish behavior in the workplace," at the same time we expect women to "carry on their traditional roles of altruistic nurturers" in other parts of their lives (25). Pillow (2004) calls this a "dual-role" expectation, and writes of how this double expectation has affected not only recent welfare policy but the schools' attitude toward teen mothers as well (218). Another question I want to ask, then, in this book, is about the schooling experiences of the young women I speak with. What was going to school like for these girls, before and after they became pregnant? What was school like after they became mothers? Were schooling experiences different for teen mothers a decade or so ago than they are today? Were schooling experiences different for middle-class young mothers than they were for young mothers who were from working-class backgrounds? And what did teachers have to say about these questions?

Where the Self Resides

Writing this book has been difficult, in part because I struggle with the discourses, the common stories, the stereotypes about teen mothers afloat in the society around us, as most people do. In telling their own stories teen mothers contend with those available fictions of female becoming as well; they work to be seen as complicated people through those discourses, and to see themselves through them, too. Some of the teachers I speak to in these pages describe the ways that stereotypes about teen mothers have affected the ways in which they work with their students as well. Pillow (2004) writes about the "overrepresented, hypervisible" teen mother who is seen only through stereotypes that produce "gaps" in society's knowledge about her (5). She asks: "How do we tell stories that do not easily fit into existing, hypervisible, narrative structures?" (6). She describes working against "structuring stories of teen mothers as feminist victim (teen mother as victim of her circumstances) or feminist victory (teen mother who overcomes the odds)"; she describes how, even as she thought she'd succeeded telling new stories about teen mothers, audiences she read for at conferences heard her stories differently, hearing those stories as organized into stereotypical narratives (6). Similarly, although not speaking directly to the stereotypes surrounding the image of the teen mother, Thomas Newkirk (1992) writes about ways educational researchers become trapped by stereotypical narratives: Case study research, he writes, tends to be deeply conservative because its very satisfaction lies in the way it aligns itself with "mythic narratives," those "deeply rooted story patterns that clearly signal to the reader the types of judgments to be made" (135). The story I tell at the beginning of this chapter, of the young teacher bewildered by the young mothers she tries to teach, most probably pleases (assuming it does) in part because it fits certain of our expectations of narratives about young teachers on their first day of school (think of Sidney Poitier's first day of school in *To Sir with Love*). You just know—partly because the first day was so bad—that the teacher will be triumphant in the end. As much as I can I want to try—as I think the young mothers in the stories I tell here are trying—to work against those mythic, conservative, hypervisible, stereotypical, and extremely available fictions.

As I've written this book I've often wondered what I'm doing, still thinking about those girls I knew so many years ago, still interested in young women who become pregnant at inconvenient times, still curious about their stories. I'd pull out folders stuffed with students' writing from 1980 and look at the blue ink of the yellowing pages students wrote for me back when I was a young teacher. I'd read those old papers, like this research paper on the problem of teenage pregnancy, by teen mother Kathy Gonzalez:

> Teenagers have a number of mental problems such as drugs, alcohol, some runaway but teenage pregnancy is quite common. An estimated four million girls aged fifteen to nineteen and an additional 400,000 thirteen- and fourteen-year olds get pregnant every year. Why do all these girls get pregnant? Most girls get pressured into having sex, others are curious as to what sex is like. Depression, feeling they need to prove themselves, family fights, are some reasons for girls having sex.

Or this personal narrative, by Joanna Huntington:

> *How I found out I was pregnant*
>
> I'll start from the beginning. I left Mike August 16 and was living with my mom at the time. Anyway I went over to my aunt's house for the weekend I wasn't feeling to great. I didn't want to eat anything and all I did was cry I just thought I was upset over Mike, so anyway I told my Aunt Sherry that I wasn't feeling to hot so I asked her if she could take me to see a doctor. So that following Monday 20th of August she took me to see Dr. Hamilton at Utah Clinic. Dr. Hamilton ran a uran test so he told us to have a seat. We waited for about 15 minutes and that seemed like forever when finally came and asked us to go into his office right then and there I knew I was pregnant I just had a feeling.

Charmed and troubled once again as I read those papers, I was sent back in time, remembering those days when I worked at the Teen Moms' Program on the second floor of the old brick Johnson High School building in that little city in Utah.

Heather, the girl who said she resented her daughter 80% of the time, was a student with whom I was particularly close. She'd stay after class to ask me about my life, to comment on my clothes, to critique my teaching ("Child Development is getting better and better, Cindy, but English still sucks"). She'd tell me about her daughter, give me recipes for macaroon-cherry-chocolate chip-coconut bars, express irritation if I was too busy to pay attention to her, and advise me about how to get a man.

One day, seeing me taking notes on some incident that had happened in Child Development class, she decided on a new task for me: "Cindy!" she said,

"You should write a story about us!"

In some ways, so many years later and about a completely different set of women in different schools, a different state, and a different time, this is that story.

Chapter 2

Feeling Poverty:
Entering the Teen Mothers' Worlds

There was something a little subversive, I thought, a little bit peculiar, about the way I was taking time off from my job every other Tuesday. Every other Tuesday, all through the spring and summer of 2003, I'd leave my comfortable gray cubicle in the new corporate offices with the fountain outside and the abstract art on the walls, my job writing scripted curriculum, my job right in the middle of Bush's *No Child Left Behind*, and drive far up north to a little community college so that I could talk to a group of "at risk" high school–aged students about how they saw themselves, as mothers, students, readers, and writers, and about how they'd experienced the traditional Midwestern schools from which they'd, sometime ago, dropped out. These girls were providing me with the material for my book; they were my "informants"—a term that made me feel like Briscoe on *Law and Order*, shaking down some puny druggie—they were my "research subjects"—a term that made me think of a scientist in a white coat studying rats—strangely, to me, they were not my students, my clients, my friends, or even, really, my responsibility.

When I'd gone off to teach at the Teen Moms' Program so long ago, my friend Dave—then a volunteer for the United Farm Workers, now a bankruptcy lawyer—had said that he admired what I was doing, and then he'd quoted Winston Churchill's old saw to me, "A man who is not radical when he is young has no heart; a man who is still radical when he is old has no head." Leaving aside the "man" part—as if gender can ever be left aside—Dave seemed to be warning me, then, that I would change. And he'd been right, too, because here I was, years later, far, far away from the teaching with which I had thought I would change the world.

I'd worked with pregnant teens in that alternative school, with poor farm boys in a traditional high school, and with refugees in a GED program. I'd read Freire and Kozol, Postman and Weingartner. I'd tried, in my young way, to use education as a means of helping those poor students move up into the middle class, up into better lives, up into a world more like the one I'd been born into, and I'd come smack up against what Barbara Tye (2000) calls the "hard truths" about the "deep structure of schooling:" Hard Truth number one: that, as Bullough states, "the race for knowledge and position is far from fair even at the starting line; most of those who get ahead even within a public school setting begin with tremendous advantages" (as quoted in Tye 2000, 32). Hard Truth number two: that, despite the truth of that last sentence, we continue to believe, as a nation, in the conventional wisdom that "the system allows the best and the brightest to rise to the top (and that they can rise from any social class)" (Tye 2000, 31). Hard Truth number three: that even the poor have bought into the American myth that "anyone can get ahead if he or she will just buckle down and work hard" (94).

That year so long ago I'd begun to experience the strange "figured world" of working-class teen mothers, a world separate from the middle-class one I lived in, one with its own rules and ideas, "peopled by the figures, characters, and types who carry out its tasks and who have styles of interacting within, distinguishable perspectives on, and orientations towards" that world (Holland et al. 1998, 51). I'd done my best by the girls I'd met, I'd complained to everyone I knew about how hard their lives were—and then I'd left teaching altogether, married, had a son, moved across the country a couple of times and finally, found work—work that used a little bit of my background in education—in an educational publishing company.

I'd worried, that first day in the back of the career room where I met the girls, about the ease with which Angel—pale and elbowy with shimmering golden-red hair—signed the consent form I pushed in front of her.

"You're not eighteen yet, so your mother has to sign it, too," I said and, in her way, her tone so cheery it always made me wonder about her intelligence, Angel said, "Oh don't worry, she'll sign it. She don't really bother about me— she's always signing whatever I shove under her nose." I'd be concerned, I thought, wouldn't I? I'd want to know who this person who was talking to my daughter was, even if my daughter were seventeen, wouldn't I? Immediately judging Angel by her accent, her paleness, her car that looked like it was held together by rubber bands, I judged her mother, too, drew up a mental picture of her: coarse, hard, neglectful. I castigated myself for those assumptions, of course, and yet I thought, as a mother, that Angel's mom must just not care about her, not as much as I care about my son.

And so I moved back into that world I had left behind, that world of the schools, where I had always felt a little bit uncertain of my actions, a little bit guilty in my judgments, a little bit anxious in my role. Wendy Luttrell (2003) writes, "at its core, education is an anxiety-provoking enterprise" (171). Luttrell cites the sociologist Jenny Shaw, who compares schools to hospitals: Both institutions organize rituals to protect their workers, Shaw says, from the feelings of grief and loss that are created by their day-to-day work. Both institutions try to keep their workers from creating "deep personal attachments" to clients; both try to minimize their workers' "feelings of helplessness"; both try to soothe these emotions by creating depersonalizing routines and encouraging workers to deny their own responsibility for the pain they see around them. Both institutions, Shaw says, in order to function, must shield workers from their constant "proximity to suffering" (as quoted in Luttrell 2003, 174).

Well, here suffering was, I thought, as I talked to one potential informant on the phone—a girl I never met—who said she didn't know if she'd be able to come in to talk to me because her boyfriend had walked out on her and she'd been going through "a whole lotta stuff," with her kids, "I mean some *serious* stuff." And here poverty was, I thought, as I took a consent form from another girl—a girl who never came back after that day—who was three-months pregnant and really needed a job and wasn't sure she'd have enough money for gas so she could get to the school to talk to me again.

Here I was, older, sadder, and not a minute wiser, I thought, back in it again.

Some Guides Along the Way

Beth Manning, an administrator at the Thomas Jefferson Learning Center, and Melinda Vane, a career counselor at the Alyssa Learning Center, helped me move back into that anxiety-provoking world of alternative high schools. The learning centers where Beth and Melinda worked both operated under the auspices of Prairie Community College, a highly regarded two-year school with centers around the state. The main site of Prairie Community College was in Bloomfield, a Midwestern city of smokestacks and layered highways, a town that was the home of two small colleges, three internationally known companies, a farm baseball team, multiple cultural and historical centers, and mansions surrounded by large gardens, as well as the area I mostly visited, where row after row of little wooden houses sat across from bleak and empty shopping malls. Bloomfield, in 2003, when I was first visiting it, was the home of about 125,000 people; its population was mostly white, with three percent black, one percent Asian and one percent Latino. I conducted research at both the Thomas Jefferson Center, which was in Bloomfield, and the Alyssa Center, which was housed in a Prairie Community College site in Alyssa, a suburb of Bloomfield. I conducted research at two alternative high schools rather than one because each had a very different clientele and I wanted to meet and work with young mothers who had varied school and life experiences.

As I tried to convince the young mothers who came in and out of the learning centers to join my book group, I often felt ill at ease. The young women I spoke with didn't seem all that comfortable either—they were edgy, or jaded, or so vulnerable that their neediness ached out from them. Most were clearly students who had somewhere expressed what schools might consider an inappropriate emotionality. They were working-class young women whose feelings—which are not necessarily individual or private things (Boler 1999)—were often not well articulated, or in line with the wishes of the powers that be. They had not let their emotions be controlled by those teachers who act for the educational establishment, as "caring police" who, Boler might say, try to manage their students' hearts (22). Beth and Melinda, watching their students from two different schools, each had a lot to say about the emotional work of teaching, about the feelings they had heard about or seen on their students' faces, about the ways in which they had learned to talk to across class differences, and about how they made sense of the sadness they saw every day.

A strong, warm, thoughtful woman in her early fifties, Beth Manning, who had been a pregnant teenager herself before a brief marriage at eighteen, had earned a degree from a local community college, then finished a BA in the social sciences. She had held jobs as an income maintenance worker for more than a decade, helping single mothers and their children coordinate requirements for work or welfare funding, housing, and daycare. She had also worked at vocational rehabilitation centers, carrying caseloads of the chronically mentally ill and "guys that were just kind of crushed by their disability and were angry and impatient about how life had turned out for them." After those years she had finished a master's degree in literacy education from a local university, then worked in refugee services and as a literacy specialist with adults who speak English as a second language. One day in 2003 she walked me through the Thomas Jefferson Learning Center, a brick elementary school building built in 1910. We passed a red, yellow, and orange mural of a genie rubbing his lamp matted on one wall, and a document listing "Jefferson's successes and failures" that hung in a glass case on another wall.

In her position as administrator at the Learning Center, Beth said, she worked with many different kinds of students:

> There's traditionally aged high school students who dropped out of school, they got bored, they wanted to go faster than they could at a traditional high school or they

also wanted to work. They tend to be really smart, the kinds of students any teacher would dream of having. . . . Then there are guys that have lost their jobs, that have gotten to a certain point without a diploma or a GED but now need to get one. There are some guys from the prison. . . . There's a significant minority of single parents, and they can be anywhere from teenage to in their early twenties and they've come back to get this missing piece. A lot of them want to go to community college. There are some second language learners, and then there are students who have been expelled. If you're expelled from your high school you can't go to your local alternative school, so they have to come here. Many of these students were expelled for possession of drugs, that's a biggie.

I spoke with Beth in depth during the years I conducted this research, and she will speak again many times in this book. Though Beth's voice is important in these pages, and though Brenda, one of the young mothers I got to know, studied at the Thomas Jefferson Learning Center, the majority of my research was conducted at the smaller learning center where Melinda worked, in Alyssa.

After a long drive behind trucks and past smokestacks and brown-and-yellow fields, I pulled into the parking lot of the Prairie Community College site in Alyssa, a Bloomfield suburb whose little downtown was lined with brick shops, like Antic Granny's Antiques and the Country Home Gift Shop, which had green awnings and potted geraniums at the stairs. Near the Alyssa Park Square, down the block from big houses with shuttered windows and wrap-around porches, across from a Presbyterian church and a mattress factory, I entered the side door to the Alyssa Learning Center. I followed college girls who hoisted backpacks and swapped lipstick and pulled out their copies of *A Separate Peace* or *Of Mice and Men*. When they turned down the hall, I went straight into the high school center, the learning center's career room. In the career room with its low gray tables, blackboard, chart about the kings and queens of England and blue sign listing varieties of careers a high school-graduate could pursue, Melinda conducted intake interviews and guided students toward proper work. A former high school English teacher, married with a high–school–aged son, Melinda worked nights to complete a degree in counseling. She described her career counseling work at the Alyssa Learning Center as her "ideal job."

Though keeping track of numbers was difficult at the Alyssa Center, a school with a shifting population that kept no records of attendance, Melinda reasoned that about 30 students came into the three rooms—two classrooms and the career room—of the school at any one day. Most of the students at this site, Melinda told me, were in their early twenties; most were fairly affluent, and all were white. Because Alyssa was a wealthy suburb, the high school in the neighboring town that most students came from was the best, and most affluent, in that town. "Our students aren't stereotypical," Melinda said. "Most people, when you say alternative school, think of juvenile delinquents, but our students aren't." As an example of this, Melinda mentioned that one of the pregnant students who had graduated from the school recently was the mayor's daughter.

At both sites curriculum was created and updated by Prairie Community College; Melinda told me that the same curriculum had been in place for the past twenty-odd years; she called those courses, "not great, but adequate. Your basic, typical high school curriculum." She said that there was not a "vast array" of different courses for students to take, and only one, family living 1 and 2, that in any way related to a teen parent's needs to learn about mothering, getting along with a new husband or boyfriend, or dealing with family stresses.

There was also little connection between either of the learning centers and the community. Melinda described one course, called career connections, to which she invited a worker from Planned Parenthood, a worker from the human relations department at a major business in the area, and a loan officer in the bank in to talk to the students about the work they did. In this course she tried to teach students life skills, Melinda said, but most other courses were taught out of a book. Most of the courses taught were ones like spelling, health, literature 1 and 2, writing, biology, or personal development.

Though both Beth and Melinda believed in the service the learning centers were providing for students for whom traditional high schools didn't work, they both also worried about the kind of education teen mothers in particular received there. The centers operated under what Melinda called a "come-and-go" system, in which students could come into the school, pull their textbooks or related worksheets from a shelf in the room, sit down at one of the long tables, and complete their studies in silence, for however long a period of time they had available at that moment. Beth told me that the centers had originally been set up for adults who wanted to finish their GEDs, but that more and more high school students were enrolling: "What does it say about how high schools are treating their students, that we've had so many more kids—high school students—coming to us these past few years?" Melinda said she worried that troubled students didn't have much chance to speak to each other, or to adults who might help them, in the site at which she worked. Beth argued that the come-and-go aspect of the school was particularly useful for teen parents, who might not have the kind of time a traditional school would require, although, she conceded, "mothers and pregnant ones are the kids that are the hardest to keep coming here."

With Beth and Melinda's help I set up a book club that met for five months, every other Tuesday, in the back of the career center where Melinda worked. I wanted to see if reading young-adult novels about teen pregnancy, talking about those books, and writing about themselves could help the teen mothers develop a kind of community through literature: I wanted to see if the teen mothers identified with the young women in the stories they read, if they learned with them or felt comforted that someone had imagined their situations well. I also wanted to see if these books could help me begin conversations about what it means to be a woman, a student, and a mother in this culture. I wanted to create a literacy group that was not narrowly focused on "functional" literacy, as so many groups for teenage parents are. The purposes of such functional literacy classes were sometimes, to my mind, tied to attempts to educate students' emotions so that, under the rules "of industrial capitalism, [they would not] set up expectations that will not be fulfilled within the society" (Boler 1999, 51). I wanted the young women in my literacy group, rather, to read in order to feed their imaginations and their "rebellious spirits" (Vargos Llosa 2001).

In my work at the educational publishing company, I was involved in defining one standard of literacy, a traditional kind of literacy in which the text holds its meaning by itself, separate from the experiences or emotions of the reader. This conception of literacy suggests that knowledge can be separated into a series of book-learned facts. This idea of literacy, with which I struggled at work, had its uses, its very narrow time and place, I believed, but I was more interested in a way of thinking about reading and writing that would help students understand the different discourses at work in the world around them and help them, as Robert Yagelski (2000) writes, "to see their connection to the broader discourses and social forces that shape their lives and to understand how [what they read and write is] inextricably linked to those ideas and forces" (180). I wondered how reading and writing about other young mothers might help the young women in my book club think critically about their own situations, and perhaps stand up against the pervasive stereotypes around them. Finally, I knew from my experience teaching at the Teen Moms' Program that simply talking to other teen mothers, hearing about other young women's experiences with motherhood, and learning practical tips about jobs or doctors or baby-rearing techniques might boost self-esteem, ease loneliness, and encourage the young mothers to build stronger identities as women and as mothers as well.

After some work, I found four teen mothers, Brenda Parker, Angel Brown, Gabriel Banks, and Casey Howard, and worked with them, collecting interviews and book club discussions on audiotape and in my notebooks, reading their written work, and just generally getting to know them, for over fifty hours during the spring and summer semesters of 2003, and then again in 2004. Each of the young women was at a different stage of mothering, each of them was white, and all were trying to finish high school. All of the women I spoke with, except Gabriel, who said she didn't care, chose the names by which they are called here.

Not Rich but Not Poor

> **Angel:** You see, on St Samuel Island, it's a really like, richy section, where everybody has these humongous houses and they have to have everything perfect in one little section. That's just how Alabama is—it's terrible. And what else you got, you got the okays, and the fairs, and the very very poors. And all of us in one little section, it's not too pretty.
>
> **Cynthia:** What were you?
>
> **Angel:** We're not a very rich family. Like we've always had what we need and then . . . we've always had clothes, nice clothes like, not very top name brands like Tommy and all that stuff, but we always had food and stuff. We're normal, average. Not rich but not poor. In the middle.

When I met with my "informants," Angel and Casey, Gabriel and Brenda, when we read young-adult novels about teen parenting together, I began to realize all I hadn't known about the lives of the poor, and I began to remember some of the things I had felt uncomfortable about the year I taught at the Teen Moms' Program. I hadn't known how awkward trying to help another person can be, how easy it is to feel self-righteous or confused or beaten down or just stymied in attempts to communicate with young people whose emphases in life, expressions of self, and ways of communicating are vastly different from your own conventional, middle-class, female ways. I hadn't known, when I was teaching at the Teen Moms' Program, how hard it is for people to change their ways, to leave a violent man, or to stop replicating relationships lived in and around when young. I hadn't known how good becoming a mother can look when everyone else you know is having a baby young, when husbands and boyfriends come and go. I hadn't known, either, about the gulf that would rise up between me and the working-poor girls I wanted to talk with, the ways in which we couldn't understand each other, the ways in which the things I assumed were true of family and school life were not real to them. Did anyone read to you when you were a child? I asked Casey, as part of my research. *Well, I lived in a foster home from the time I was five until the trial with my father—my real father, not the first or second stepfather—so there wasn't that much time for reading.* What does your mom think about your switching schools so much? I asked Angel, who described her moves from town to town, from home to boyfriend's house, to apartment. *She works two-and-a-half jobs, she doesn't really care where I go to school, as long as I go. The baby? Oh man, was she pissed when I first told her, but she's a happy grandma now.*

When we read one of the novels together, I asked the girls what they thought about the way the teen mother is described, living as she does, the dishes in the sink, the cobwebs, the cockroaches scuttling across her kitchen. Were they offended by this stereotypical picture of the slovenly mother, the impoverished teen parent? Well, "I know a lot about cockroaches," said Angel, "You can't get away from 'em in Alabama."

"They were—in your house?" I hear the incredulity in my voice and want to kick myself.

"In the trailer, yeah. Outside and on the ground, everywhere. I don't know if they were in restaurants too, I don't eat out too much, huh. I had to live with cockroaches for twelve years, when I was living with my grandma in her trailer. There are a lot of cockroaches in Alabama."

And then, while I was trying to reconcile myself to the idea that though she lived in a trailer, Angel still did not consider herself one of the "very very poors," but "in the middle," she added, unprompted, "I've always lived around a lot of blacks. I'm not saying—'cause I'm not prejudiced, I've had black friends but—they aren't too clean, I don't think, not too many of them care too much about being clean."

A Great Shining Moment

Up a steep flight of stairs in a rickety blue-and-yellow house I met a young woman I'll call Juliette Baldwin, who for over fifteen years had been a counselor and director of the Youth Services Center, a program that provided counseling, education, and respite care for troubled pregnant and parenting teens and their children. I had learned, in my conversations with Angel, some things that bewildered me about myself, my ignorance, and my motivations. I wondered if Juliette, who worked with the poorest and most unsettled teen mothers, could help me answer some of my questions about emotions in the classroom, about teaching and helping, and about the barriers that differences in socioeconomic class can produce.

But when I found Juliette in her office, I didn't ask her about how she felt as she worked with troubled teen mothers. I didn't ask her how she talked to her clients across that chasm of class I'd discovered between myself and Angel, how she had become empathetic to these young women or ways in which what she had studied in school had or hadn't prepared her for the suffering she saw daily. I didn't ask her whether our society's pervasive blame-the-victim discourse around poverty affected her relationships with clients, or how she worked against that discourse in her mind. I didn't ask her how she managed to keep on going in the kind of work that I had left so long ago; I didn't ask how she sustained hope or how she nourished her radical heart. Instead I talked to her about the intersection between poverty and teenage pregnancy: Why did some kids give birth and keep their children, when birth control and abortion were so readily available, and why did those girls who raised their children so often seem to be poor?

"Kids who choose to parent are kids who come from disadvantaged homes," said Juliette, without nuance or hesitation. She sat at her wooden desk in her cluttered office, next to a bookcase stuffed with paperbacks—*The Courage to Heal* and *Your Child's Self Esteem* and *Young, Poor, and Pregnant*—near a box filled with bright blue-and-red plastic trucks and counting rings and little cups, in front of a board plastered with photographs of African American and Asian and white and Hispanic babies and toddlers. Over the bulletin board was a familiar poster that read, "One hundred years from now it will not matter how big my house was or what kind of car I drove. . . ." Outside I heard someone wearing flip-flops padding by, I heard soft voices talking, and a baby in the nursery across the hall wailing. Juliette said,

> Many of the kids I work with have grown up quickly. They have had to care for a sibling because the parent has mental health problems or substance abuse problems, so they feel like they're adults, and I've heard them say, well, if I have to take care of my brother then I might as well take care of my own child. Oftentimes kids who get pregnant and are choosing to parent are kids whose families haven't helped them establish lifelong goals and their goal becomes to be a parent. They don't have this vision, I'm going to go to college and I'm going to become a doctor or a social worker or a teacher. That's not something they've lived with in their lives; that doesn't feel like an attainable goal, but being a parent does.
>
> So that's part of it, having a child will help them feel loved and they can love their children and their children will love them back, because these kids often times haven't

received that in their own lives and so parenting often becomes their identity. The kids I see aren't active in athletics, they don't do music, they're not involved in school. They have a pretty narrow focus about what life is. Many of our folks have borderline personality disorder—folks who have suffered trauma in their childhood, sexual abuse in particular, suffer from borderline personality disorder. Those folks can be real trying to work with, real crisis-oriented folks, and unless you work to get past some of their traumas they're not going to be very good parents. But also, for kids who come from pretty bleak backgrounds, having a new baby is really exciting. It was for me, too, it was the highlight of my life. ("For me, too,'" I said to Juliette). It's a pretty great shining moment in an otherwise bleak life, for these kids. And that's the bottom line: the girls who become teen parents, the ones who come here, have led some pretty crummy lives.

Ill at Ease

So, according to Juliette Baldwin, part of my awkwardness as I tried to get to know Casey, Angel, Brenda, and Gabriel could have been caused by their difficulty in trusting, based on traumas that had occurred in their lives. But I was sure there was something else, too; I was sure some of my awkwardness was related to class-based expectations and ways of expressing ourselves.

When he worked as a minister with the poor, the writer Garret Keizer (2004) says he often felt like a dupe, as if he were being used by the people he was trying to help, being lied to. Me, too: I felt manipulated often when I was reading and talking with Angel. Partly, it was that Angel's needs seemed so great. How could I fulfill, as she seemed to expect me to, even a portion of the educational, emotional, physical, and spiritual needs she expressed to me? Sometimes she irritated me by correcting me, or showing that she knew more than I did ("You never heard of the patch?"); sometimes she would embarrass me by talking about partying in a detailed way. Sometimes I felt manipulated by her because she just didn't show up: I brought her a pamphlet on the cycle of domestic abuse, thinking it might help her think about her relationship with her boyfriend, and she didn't come, didn't call; I brought back a library book I'd borrowed from her and, though I waited an hour or so, she never walked through the career center door. Maybe, partly, I felt manipulated by Angel because I have, as Keizer suggests many of us have, "what might be called a cynic or sucker response to human need": "our instinct is to act as if these are our only alternatives" (23), turning a cold shoulder or being a soft touch.

I don't know if Wendy Luttrell (2003) has read Garret Keizer's work but she speaks to much of what he says when she describes how one of the teen mothers she worked with had "disavowed feelings of loss and sorrow as part of her version of hard, protective, individualism, her tough stance toward life" (162). Luttrell believes that the reason this young woman developed her hard persona was "tied to social, structural forces of inequality." When she notices one teen mother making an angry gesture at her, Luttrell, a middle-class white woman, wonders about the complexity of her relationship with this working-class black student. Luttrell writes that she needs to think through her own "unexamined assumptions about [this student's] 'neediness' and my desire to 'help'" and then writes about the "emotional politics" (159) of class, gender, and race in the United States:

> One lesson I take from this encounter is that class-and-family-based patterns of protecting working class and poor children against hardship . . . are bound up in complex maternal-child relationships that engender mixed feelings of love, hate, dependence, and gratitude (on the part of the positioned "child" and on the part of the positioned "mother.") These feelings enter into cross-class and cross-race relationships between girls and women, . . . particularly those relationships related to care and power—teacher-student; nurse-patient; therapist-client; social-worker-client; researcher–researched. (159)

Often my uneasiness with the markers of class Angel brought with her—her slightly washed-out clothes, her disorganized family life, her lack of connection to any institutions—and my discomfort with our differences, meant that I didn't leave myself open enough to her talk. I would come away from our conversations drained and realizing that I hadn't been able to take in what she told me, hadn't been able to ask questions, hadn't challenged her unbelievable statements or pushed for interpretation. I would have missed all those hesitations, halting beginnings, dangling sentences, and changes in direction that suggest that much is being held back, unsaid.

Just Trying to Get By

Sometime after my conversation with Juliette, I visited Beth at the Thomas Jefferson Learning Center. I wondered how she would answer some of the questions my conversations with the women in the Alyssa Learning Center had brought up: Did she have difficulties empathizing across class differences? Was she confused by her own need to "help," and by her students' reactions to that need? Did she have trouble, sometimes, understanding the worlds her students came from? How did she nurture her radical heart?

As I drove through town toward the Jefferson Learning Center I thought about how enamored we are in this country with the idea of individualism.

Sharon Hays (2003) explains that our "demonization" of poor mothers is closely connected to our belief in individualism. "If people become poor, if they find themselves seeking aid at the welfare office, we say, it must be because of something they, as individuals, did or did not do. The cultural power of this analysis cannot be overestimated" (125). I knew that though I didn't intellectually believe that the poor could pull themselves up by their bootstraps, an unconscious part of myself was influenced by the individualistic discourse which every American breathes in daily. I knew that this belief made it more difficult for me to act with compassion, even with understanding, of the young women I worked with, even though I wanted to be understanding and compassionate.

In *Upheavals of Thought,* Martha Nussbaum (2001) paraphrases Aristotle, saying that "the first cognitive requirement of compassion is a belief or appraisal that the suffering is serious rather than trivial. The second is the belief that the person does not deserve the suffering. The third is the belief that the possibilities of the person who experiences the emotion are similar to those of the sufferer" (307). Many Americans may believe that having a child young is a serious "suffering," but most would continue to believe that that young woman has brought the suffering on herself, and most would not believe that they could find themselves in a position similar to the young mother. I wondered what Beth, who had worked with the working poor for so long, would have to say about this.

When I met Beth in her glassed-in office with its jade plants and photographs of her husband, her physicist son, and her white Siberian husky, she was upset because the night before she had been threatened by a "big, muscular" 28-year old Hispanic student after hours at the center. Later she had learned ("I should have been told this before") that the student had "a whole lot of stuff in his background that was pretty scary. Arrests, violent actions, domestic abuse charges."

Because the security system designed to help teachers at night had failed and no one had come to her aid, she was shaken and uncertain of the value of continuing on at that school. ("I felt pretty angry, not so much at him, but at being in a position where anybody can walk in and treat you like that and you have no resources.")

Still, Beth spoke with a respect for the people she worked with that was palpable. "What I try to offer is what they're looking for. It's not about me, it's about what they need. I think it's a matter of, you're a human being, I'm going to meet you with respect and whatever you're doing in your life is your business. I try to act that way even if I'm talking to a 16-year-old." Most of her students at Thomas Jefferson were among the working poor, Beth said; they were raising children alone or working all day.

> About ninety-nine percent of our kids are very focused. They land at Thomas Jefferson because they've made up their minds to have a better life. Sometimes they have to drop out for a while, you know, the guys say, "I had to spend a little time in jail," or "I got behind on my child support," but they come back. It's really cool to see how they come back, it's cool to work with so many focused, goal-oriented people.

> I think there are a lot of teen moms at our center that go under the radar screen. They're like I was, they don't need real extensive services, they might need welfare for a while or daycare but not mental health counseling and the kind of desperate help the folks at the Youth Services Center need. They come here because they can come to school, do their work, and go home to their children on their own schedule. And nobody bothers them. We don't handle girls' sexuality well, as a whole society I think we don't.

Beth agreed with me that it was probably easier for her to get along with most of her students than it was for teachers who had not had her experiences, because she had been a single mother for over a decade, had been on and off a welfare during those years, and remembered what it was like to be "driving a car that's falling apart, and scrambling to find daycare." She said she told her students about her time being a young, single mom, so her students knew she could empathize with them. "I tell them, oh yeah, they know. They're just trying to get by, like I did." In a story about one student, Beth pointed out, with some anger, how common it is in our society to associate wealth with moral goodness:

> One of our pregnant students comes from a, quotes, good family, which I think is a meaningless term, but you know how people will talk like this, Susan comes from such a good family! And then she does this! Susan's parents told her, at the age of 16, that getting pregnant was her own damn fault, so she had to move out and raise the kid on her own. She made her bed, she had to lie in it, her parents said. And this is a 'good family'! . . . I think by 'good family' they mean comfortably middle class, that's part of what some people think it means to be a good family, to be well-off. And that was the way they treated their daughter. To have that kind of . . . harshness . . . I know this is going to sound weird to say but I think you're going to have to pay for that, somewhere, in your life, I do. To put that kind of harshness and judgment on people, I don't think you have that right.

Beth clearly believed the "suffering" of having a child young and unwed was "serious rather than trivial," she believed that Susan did not deserve the suffering of being abandoned by her parents, and she clearly could see herself being in the same kind of trouble as Susan. All of this helped her to be compassionate. Unlike Susan's parents, Beth believed that "any of us could make a mistake, any of us could go off that path, at any moment."

But Beth doubted whether empathy could go very far across some differences: "I've seen teachers who know what it is to be poor, but they've pulled themselves up, and they don't see why these kids don't, they think they're just lazy." Although most of the teachers she worked with were wonderful, Beth thought that some didn't allow for differences of expression, some of which were related to differences in socioeconomic class. She described teachers who giggled when they met a working-class female student who had "butch" hair and was dressed in "tough" clothes:

> The teachers didn't know how to treat her because she didn't follow this very traditionally gendered approach to her appearance—she threw them for a loop. The guys come in looking alternative—spikes around the neck, and a whole lot of piercings, and a lot of girls with piercings too, but you know with long hair, not with the butch cut. I've noticed that the staff responds better to young women who are pretty, following that traditional presentation of self, although they draw a line there, too. We had a woman who came in looking like she'd just gotten off the street hooking, you know, the chest and the heels, looking like she'd been in business that evening. Nobody liked that! My staff responds more easily to the cute ones, the nice ones, the sweet ones. Even Brenda, who you're working with, they find too abrupt, direct, pretty working class. She has an edge, and the teachers here don't like that.

I wondered about what Megan Boler (1999) calls our "socially determined habits of inscribed inattention" (17), of the importance of what we choose to notice, based on our own fears, personal history, or unacknowledged beliefs about gender or class differences. Beth herself was more open to the varied ways her students chose to express their gendered selves, and their varied, perhaps class-based, ways of expressing emotions, than the teachers she worked with were. Still, Beth would agree with Boler, who writes, in a critique of Louise Rosenblatt's idea that reading can help teach empathy, that she doesn't have much faith in people's capacity to imagine what is "really happening" to others: "To judge what 'others need in order to flourish' is an exceptionally complicated proposition not easily assumed in our cultures of difference" (115).

"Well, yeah," Beth said, "it's complicated." She said,

> I think empathy is something that's got to be close to impossible, because it means you

have to have infinite patience. We're not infinitely patient and infinitely good. But listen, I don't work with these girls, these guys, because it makes me feel better about myself to be doing that, I don't do it because I'm trying to be compassionate or good. . . . I just like these folks. They've had tough times, and I think I can understand, because I've been there, but imagination . . . well, sure, there's only so far my imagination can go.

Sharing the Same Guard

Later, as I went through my day at work, I still wondered why Angel had said that she was not one of the "fairs, the okays, or the very very poors" but "in the middle." Surely Angel was expressing that American belief in a classless society, that belief that to consider oneself "in the middle" is to consider oneself normal, approved (Brantlinger 2003). Surely it was partly because she was talking to me—so clearly middle class in my dress, my language, and my assumptions—that made her use that phrase. Other older and more confident young women I spoke to for this study described themselves as "working class," and, when asked that question, some, like Casey, answered, "It's complicated. I've been living on my own since I was fifteen," thereby not exactly answering my question but speaking more to the complexity of how we define class than Angel did.

Beth described with some anger her experience speaking with people who had not had the experiences she'd had working with working-class students:

For all my life I've worked with people who are working their buns off. They're just trying to make the pieces fit so they can have a good life. And they're really aware, and that's one thing that maybe other people don't understand, that these single moms know how much they're judged. They know it inside out. They know they're lumped together and talked about like, why are you having another kid? I know a lot of young women who are very articulate about their situations. For whatever reasons, they became parents too young and it's not like 'Oh, duh, really? Did I?' They know they became parents too young and that's one reason they're back at school. They've had to be articulate from such a young age that they've learned how to talk about what they need and where they're going and—they're not *dumb*, not by a long shot. I lose patience with those people who can't empathize with these girls. Most of those people have never worked with people who are on aid or are single parents or haven't got a high school diploma. I don't know where those people get their information but they're not dealing with reality.

I agreed with Beth. I found it painful and sometimes confusing to be around Angel and Casey and Brenda, to hear their vulnerabilities, to see my own mistakes with them, to see them trying hard to explain what their lives were like to me and to see myself unable to quite get it. I felt awkward speaking to Casey who remembered,

> When Christmas comes around they kind of, on the news they'll show, basically show the poor kids, they go and see Santa, I don't remember what building that is downtown, but Santa will give them a gift. And—I sat down and I told the kids, you know when I was 6 years old all I got was one gift and it was the cheapest gift ever but it was my favorite gift and it was the only gift I got that year. It always brings back memories.

It was wonderful, and also a little confusing, to meet with Brenda in the Thomas Jefferson Learning Center, to hear her explain why she was giving up the baby she was soon to have. Imagine feeling, at twenty-two, that you have to make the kind of choice she had made:

> I can't handle another baby, financially or emotionally, because I'm already going through too much as it is with my three. I mean I just imagine going to the doctor's office with my bad boy and then trying to take care of the stroller and the diapers and all my stuff and then still carrying a newborn and keeping my eyes on the twins, too. I just can't handle it. Plus, I don't need one more if I'm going to make us a good living.

It was inspiring to hear about her plans for her own future: "I really liked the nurses at the ER. I don't know, I just always wanted—blood's never bothered me. And I really want to be a nurse but that takes four years so I'll have to wait and just be an LPN for a while. That's mostly wiping kid's butts but I got to pay the price. I wipe my own kids' butts; I guess I can wipe somebody else's." Brenda, who said she'd gotten the job she had now back when she was "flat as a board," and made a pitch for another position on her cell phone in the middle of our first conversation, described some recent hard times to me:

> All of a sudden—boom! I didn't have no income coming in, no food stamp money, nothing. My worker sent me that paper that said I needed to have proof from Work Quick because the last place I worked at was Work Quick. I had to have proof from them that I was not working. All right, she gave that to me on the twenty-seventh of March. All right, now twenty-eight, twenty-nine, thirty and thirty-one and the thirty-one was on Monday, so anyway Work Quick, it takes like two weeks for them to fax that stuff over to the DHS. I tried to tell her it takes two weeks. What are me and the kids going to do for food for that two weeks? Well, I told you, she said. I said, no, you didn't. At the end of the month you sent me a letter, at the end of the month, you didn't ask for no verification and now all of a sudden you pull this stuff on me! It was on a Friday that I got it. I was like, why are you doing this? I was stressed out for a

whole week. I finally got everything the first week of April but I had to keep calling the light bill because they threatened to shut off my lights and I needed to pay my water at the beginning of the month. I kept trying to tell them it's not my fault it's my worker. She let me know at the end of the month, if she would of let me know at the middle of the month I could of—I had only like two days to get everything in and it didn't work out but my mom, my mom does help me every now and then. When that situation came up she did help me with food. She works at Wal-Mart. We have a pretty good relationship now. She has changed.

When I spoke with Brenda I saw what Beth meant when she said, "these girls, they're not dumb," and, "I can think of a lot of young mothers who are really articulate about their situations."

When I talked with Brenda also, though, I often felt some of the guilt that Dimen (1994) refers to the sense of "fraudulence and looming loss" (as quoted in Luttrell 2003, 87) that middle-class people can feel when working with poor and working-class people. It can be difficult, writes Luttrell (2003), to get over the discomfort a middle-class person might feel about "two distinct class-based structures of feeling" (88). I also wondered, in speaking to these girls, about the psychic costs of growing up poor—the psychic costs of living hand-to-mouth were certainly evident in Brenda's stories—and about what Walkerdine (1997) calls the "patterns of defenses produced in family practices which are about avoiding anxiety and living in a very dangerous world" (as quoted in Luttrell 2003, 157).

Beth didn't seem to pay much attention to the kind of internal worry I experienced, if she had it; when I asked her if she saw herself as "saving" or "helping" the people she worked with she said,

> I don't think that I have ever thought of myself that way. I think instead of the phrase Karen Armstrong uses—'practical compassion.' You do your best to serve people respectfully, treat them straight, and that's about it. We were just providing rightful benefits. I think the more accurate ethic behind a lot of my co-workers was a belief in some form of justness in a society. Not that any of us ever talked that way—we all had pretty awful senses of humor that sounded a bit twisted to anyone on the outside.

Often, as I drove back to the educational publishing company from the learning center where I talked and read with Angel, Brenda, and Casey, religious metaphors flowed into my mind. In his book about his life as a teacher, *No Place but Here*, Garret Keizer (1988), complaining that so many of our educational metaphors are ones of sports or war or business, of the cop on the beat or the administrator becoming more efficient, suggests that a religious metaphor for what the teacher does might be more helpful. Why not think of the teacher as the pastor of his flock rather than the coach of his team, Keizer suggests. If metaphors matter, if the metaphor suggests that which we measure ourselves against, how much better to measure oneself against the preacher rather than the policeman (137).

Deborah Hicks (2002) writes that she finds teachers who work with poor and working-class students often blame the parents, the students themselves, or the community in which they live. "What has to occur for things to change is not simply an intellectual shift, so that teachers have more information," she writes. "Rather, change also has to entail a moral shift, a willingness to open oneself up to the possibility of *seeing* those who differ from us. This is very hard work, but work that lies at the heart of teaching" (152).

I was in the middle of my life, in between one world—the world of business, and cubicles, a world of ready-to-buy curricula, concerns about students' "socioeconomic status" and the company's bottom line, and another—the world of alternative schools where young mothers drove rattletrap cars and filled out worksheets and tried to explain themselves to middle-aged researchers. I was in the middle, between one idea of what literacy, what knowledge was— an accumulation of book-learned facts that could be memorized for a test— and another idea, that said literacy is an interconnected sense of a widening conversation between different voices in the world. I was in the middle, in my relationships with these young women, in between an image of who I wanted to be—someone more like Beth—and who I was, the nervous, emotionally raw new researcher. I wasn't really sure if, in doing this work, I was "gawking at someone's difficulties" or, as I would rather be, sitting next to them in hard times, keeping watch with them, and, as Keizer (2004) says, "sharing the same guard" (244). I wasn't sure whether the teachers who worked with these young women, and the writers who wrote the books we would read together, weren't using these young women in some way, too, using these young women's "otherness" to prove their own value. I was in the middle between a fascination and a familiarity with the world of these teen mothers and an almost instinctive recoiling from it, a recoiling these young women surely must have sensed in me. Just beginning, old to the young women I spoke with and yet once again too vulnerable, too new, I gathered up my books and my pencils, my notepads and my recording equipment and tapes, collected my questions and my anxieties, and once again, drove home.

Poor Girls, Reading, and Me

It was the children's books, I'm tempted to think, which taught me such an early and sentimental concern for the poor. All of those stories I lived in as a child—*Racketty-Packetty House*, in which the dolls in their rags and tatters happily served each other five courses at supper, each course consisting entirely of turnips; *Little Women*, in which Jo sighed, "It's so dreadful to be poor!" with a kind of contentment, by the fireplace on the very first page; *All of a Kind Family*, in which Papa thought, "So much money spent on a fancy cup and saucer that I could just as well do without," when his daughters bought him a birthday present—all of those books convinced me, growing up in New Haven, Connecticut, in the affluent 1960s, that to be Poor was very closely aligned with being Blessed.

Being poor, one had a chance of being noble in a way that one had no opportunity for, when one was a successful professor's daughter. Being poor, one could shoulder one's burdens without complaint. Being poor, like Dan, the bad boy with the heart of gold in *Little Men*, or like Polly, who doesn't wear fashionable clothes in *An Old Fashioned Girl*, would help one grow closer to God, it was clear, become more immediately redeemable, and—inevitably—wiser than the rich. Think of all that Heidi taught Clara.

Though reality seemed less—real—to me than those books I read (Atwell-Vasey 1998, 131), I knew reality was different from the books. Any evidence of class differences I saw around me when I was a child was—well, discomforting. I disliked the K-Mart dresses some of the black girls in school wore, and I noticed with disdain that a friend of mine came to school wearing dresses that were too short for her, and flip-flops instead of real shoes. I didn't like Orange Street, where Beverly Manzi, my friend, and Rudy Abrams, my nemesis, lived in apartments, different from the grand old houses—shabby but dignified—in which most of the kids I knew lived. The working-class people I knew, I thought—Italians and Poles, those Manzis and Riggios, those Pollaks and Snigeroviches and Jacksons—weren't the *real* poor. The real poor I invested with sentimentality, with romance: the real poor were somehow, in my mind, as they were portrayed on the leaves of the Victorian children's books I read,

Other from me, tinged with a Beauty that few people I knew in real life could ever quite acquire.

But I realized it was wrong to want to *be* poor, so somewhere toward the end of elementary school I switched goals: I would become a Helper of the Poor. I wanted to be an orphan, like Pollyanna, playing the Glad Game even though my life was Tough, walking around with my hands behind my back and a big bow in my hair, cheering up all the lonely old people in town. All those orange-backed little biographies on the bookshelves in Miss Sandy Shrubs's fifth-grade classroom—with names like *Jane Addams: Girl Reformer*; *Molly Pitcher: Young Patriot*, or *Florence Nightingale: Songbird for the Sick*—convinced me that in order to have a life of worth it was necessary that I join that female procession of Fixers, to work with the mothers and the children that Marmee so often went out into the streets to serve, to join with Annie Sullivan as she brought Helen Keller into light and language. I wanted to possess that passion, that empathy, that freedom from guilt, that peace those women seemed to share. The last words of the biography of Anne Sullivan I read and reread certainly promised peace to a stormy little girl: "The silent storm within her was stilled at last."

Who knew what poverty was really like, outside of Victorian children's books? Not me. But it was this image of poverty as something we were put here on Earth to rid the world of, this image of poverty as a place where souls struggled with a kind of shimmer that was not present in my immediate life, and this picture of myself as a kind and helpful woman, a sort of savior, that led me, as it has led so many others, to become a teacher.

Chapter 3

Life Stories:
Listening to Teen Mothers' Lives

I'm just saying to these pregnant girls, weigh out the pros and cons. 'Cause I heard one story that was in Bingtown somewhere? A girl left her baby by the side of the road? I'm like, oh my goodness. And there was one mother down in Mississippi or Florida that watched her kids drown in the car. She drove her kids out into the river and watched them drown.

That's just sick. I mean she said it was postpartum depression but that's no excuse. I had postpartum depression after my twins and all I did was cry. I didn't cry saying, I hate my kids. You're just emotional, you're not like, well I think I'm going to drive my kids off into the river. I think she just didn't want to take responsibility. But that's why I have the adoption set up. There's plenty of people that would have adopted that lady's kids. There was a baby, a two-year-old, I think, and three of them in the car.

Seems like people would be glad I'm giving this next one up for adoption, seeing on how all these mothers keep killing their kids. That's just sad. If you don't want your child there is another family out there that can't have children that will be in love with your child.

—Brenda

When I talked to the young women I interviewed for this book, layered into the stories they told—of fights with their mothers, difficulties with men, and the ways they thought through how they'd raise their children—there was another story, one more important than the rest, more important than the one—about literacy, about school—that I wanted the young women to tell. This story was about "weighing out the pros and cons"; about what was important in life, what was right to do and wrong to overlook. It was about growing up poor, struggling in school and trying to become a person, about marriage and mothering and being a daughter. It was also a story about love.

Brenda

"I want to be somebody"

The first day I met her, one afternoon in Beth Manning's office at the Thomas Jefferson Center, Brenda Parker told me that at school she had always been "one of them ones that blended into the wall." I had a hard time believing it—the edgy, strong, articulate woman with her black hair pulled back into one long braid down her back, a dark blue windbreaker ballooning out behind her, blue jeans unbuttoned around her slightly pouting belly—didn't seem like anyone who could ever be ignored.

Twenty-two, still married to, though no longer living with, the African American father of her children—one six-year-old and four-year-old twins—Brenda was the oldest of the four young mothers I got to know. When I asked her to choose two words that described her she said, "integrity, because I don't cheat and I don't lie," and "intimate, 'cause I'm intimate with my kids."

Brenda spoke fiercely, with anger and humor. She reminded me of the poor women Lisa Dodson (1998) describes as having to have "hearts of iron" to get ahead, women who struggle to climb out of poverty, earn an education, and build good lives for themselves and their children. Dodson suggests that there's a "buried history" (152), a positive story that's not told often enough, about poor women like Brenda moving off of welfare. She suggests that it is not until women are well into their twenties—often older than Brenda—that they develop enough sense of self to leave destructive relationships and seek out institutions that might help them (147). Dodson also emphasizes the importance of "real opportunity and practical help" (150) that moves beyond political rhetoric, help from places, perhaps, like the Thomas Jefferson Learning Center, where poor women can be respected and understood, and where they can see other women like themselves getting job training, high school diplomas, and connections to community colleges or mental health counseling (150).

When she introduced me to her, Beth Manning described Brenda as "one of the most determined people I've ever met." "She's driven," Beth said (a word, I reflected, that even now we don't often use positively about women), "She's finished whole classes in a few weeks, reading entire textbooks and taking chapter tests every other day. She's articulate, too. She'll tell you what it's like to be a mother trying to finish high school. . . . She is so sharp!"

Brenda wanted to graduate from high school and go to community college, to become a licensed practical nurse. "I want to make something of myself," she said, "I'm not going be one of them teenyboppers working at McDonald's every day. I want to be somebody."
Brenda described how it had been:

> From August until January I was doing school here at Jefferson until two o'clock, and I was doing a second shift job at the same time. At Big Chief. And I started work at three and I did not get done until two in the morning. And they were doing a lot of overtime and the temps, when you're a temp, you don't get paid that much overtime,

not as much as the actual workers, so they keep the temps longer and they always kept me longer. I tried to tell the boss-man I got to go to school, I got to pick up my kids which—Big Chief is over here on Y Street, I had to go clear out to Alyssa to pick up my kids. If I got off at two in the morning I had to worry about picking them up and bringing them back here in the middle of the night. And then, at three o'clock I'd be putting them to bed and getting myself some sleep and then getting them up at six o'clock in the morning because they got to be at school at seven. And in between that time I was doing homework. Trying to do my homework.

And then I found out I was pregnant again—in November my husband came back in the house and tried to, you know, work things out. We weren't doing nothing but arguing all the time and then in December he left because he didn't want me to go to school. He said I should give up school, and just work day shifts and skip school. I didn't want to stop school, I wanted to get my high school diploma! I wanted to go to college!

Brenda laughed—loud!—when she described all the stupid jobs she'd had ("I was packing fruit roll-ups!") and how bad the work itself was ("You do the same thing over and over, a 12-hour shift standing in the same spot like a zombie, and you get breaks, but only enough to grab a cigarette"). She was wise to the ways the powers that be used her, describing how the "boss-man" was always "pulling stuff on me." She patiently guided me through the lists of government agencies she'd had to deal with, knowing that I was too middle class to be familiar with the acronyms. When I asked her why she wanted to be a nurse she grinned and said, "I've always liked bluuud," and then corrected herself, giving the gender-appropriate response, "No, no, I really want to help people."

"He don't like my assertiveness now"

In bits and pieces, Brenda told me the story of her life, with what she considered the most important parts—her marriage, her struggles with her children, and her work to attain an education—getting most emphasis. She told a story of a family made chaotic by poverty, of a mother who would take her out of school for no reason and a father who was accused of "doing something to one of his other kids," and so wasn't around very much. School had been difficult for her, and she had a lot to say about that:

I always had problems reading in school, matter of fact I flunked first grade because of reading. Because I couldn't put my words together. They found that out after I wasn't getting things done in first grade. So they held me back a year and put me in some special helping class. And I still to this day remember getting made fun of from getting held back. I seriously think it was the school's fault. They could of paid more attention. I mean if you could tell I wasn't getting good grades on none of my school work from the get-go.

As all children do, Brenda had presented her "unguarded self" to a new set of adults who, she was told, held "knowledge and authority" (Dodson 1998, 187). Because she felt something untrue in how they saw her she fought against these adults, and against her peers who she felt ostracized her because of her shabby clothes, ungrammatical talk, and, perhaps, her hard, working-class edge. "I signed up for clubs, I tried 'em, but those preppies they wouldn't let me in," she said of junior high. She got into fights with other girls in high school, and because of those fights, and perhaps the inappropriate emotionality that they expressed, she was suspended. She tried to run away from home but her mother "sent the cops after me." For part of high school she moved or was moved into a "treatment home."

> We would go to school, and we'd get made fun of because we were in the treatment home, see, that's just another clique. But at the treatment home at least they made me do my homework. They gave me structure, and I needed that structure. But I quit in tenth grade.

She married early ("I was seventeen. I was in *looove*") and had a baby immediately ("I just pop 'em out"). She described the marriage's ups and downs:

> We broke up, me and my husband separated. He left me and my son out in Las Vegas six months pregnant with the twins and only five dollars and no relatives out there or nothing. So I called my relatives, crying, and they got a bus ticket for me 'cause I still hadn't had the twins yet and they told me I wasn't supposed to travel, but I wasn't about to be out there in Las Vegas when I couldn't go nowhere. So I came back here from Vegas, pregnant with the twins and with my son, and by then it had been about a year and a half since I saw my mom. I was trying to give her a second chance. I had the twins and she was there for the delivery and I named my daughter after her because she supposedly had changed and all that blah blah blah.

This story seemed to be a central one, one that narrative researchers Elinor Ochs and Lisa Capps (2001) would call a "turning point" (215) in the plot of Brenda's life, in which the main character "undergoes a transformation of identity (215)," beginning to see herself as having some agency, and falling upon resources other than the ones her husband provided. Brenda described herself as loyal, though, and as trying to work it out with her husband:

He's a trucker, and by then he had his own truck, and he decided why don't we go over the road in the truck. I was like all willing, I tried it, but I was going out of my mind because I was taking care of the kids—three kids under four—in a semi truck! I mean trying to keep them quiet going across the scales and stuff so because none of us had riders' passages and trying to make a truck into some kind of home and we did that as long as I could stand it.

She described past and current frustrations with her husband ("It was mental, never physical abuse"). She explained why she still had an off-and-on relationship with him ("He's the father of my babies!").

When I asked her about her current reading, Brenda said she read mostly when she put her three children to bed. Each night she read them

Thomas the train books and Scooby doo and Barbie books. Each one of them has their own books that they want to read at night. One kid'll sit down and listen to one book and then the next one says, oh, I didn't want that book, so I've got to read another book, so basically, I'm doing my reading with my kids. I don't get no special sit-down-on-my-own-and-read time.

She'd learned a lot at the Thomas Jefferson Learning Center, reading "science books cause I'm taking a science class now" and, in her composition class, "doing a journal every day," which was hard because she couldn't think of much to say beyond recounting the events that had occurred. The teachers at the Thomas Jefferson Learning Center, and Beth in particular, had helped her "navigate" between her mothering work at home, her money-earning work, and her school work.

Over time, she had developed more instincts for self-preservation. She described how the Thomas Jefferson Learning Center had helped her become more precious to herself:

I used to—when my husband and I first got together until the last time we broke up, it was like he would say jump and I'd say how high? I was so dependent on him, where I'd listen to what he would say. If I went over to my girlfriend's house, he'd say, what are you, lesbian? We just wanted to talk girl talk, you know, like with a sister, about hair and clothes and stuff and he said we were lesbians! He was controlling. But I stuck by him, even after he left me there in Las Vegas. He was my first love and I had my kids by him so automatically I was like, all right, I'll take you back, but now, I got stronger and more independent. Partly because of school and these people here at this school they will help you, they will navigate with you. Partly just being on my own, raising three kids on my own I figure I know some things. I'm more assertive. He doesn't want me to go to college because I think he's scared that if I got better than him I wouldn't put up with none of his crap anymore. He don't like my assertiveness now.

Angel

"I know all about that"

Tall, thin, with long golden-red hair and a thick Alabama accent, seventeen-year-old Angel Brown slammed into the Alyssa Learning Center late the day I first met her, and already talking. "I had trouble with my vehicle," she said, her accent so thick I could hardly understand her, "You the one who wants to talk to pregnant girls? You studying teen pregnancy? Well, I know all about that."

Angel was from Stonesville, a town of about 4,000, a place that was the home of a maximum security prison and not much else. The prison's website shows the white stone Gothic administration building against a blue sky, and lighted up at night; the five-ton stone lions guarding the steps at the entrance of the penitentiary, the flower beds along the curving driveway. The website asks you to "enjoy!" your visit to the penitentiary museum, and promises photos of famous criminals, including a nine-year old lifer. You can see the word *Hope* imprinted on a tin floor plate at the entrance to Living Unit D.

Angel and her mother moved from Alabama, where they had lived in a cockroach-filled trailer with her grandmother, to a town near Stonesville and then to Stonesville itself, when her father was moved to the prison there. Many of the people in town were wives, girlfriends, and mothers who had moved to the town to be close to family who were doing time. When I told Beth Manning that Angel said she loved it in Stonesville, Beth said, "Wow. That says a lot about her. That's a really tough town, really a terrible town. She must be a really vulnerable kid."

Angel had moved from Alabama when she was twelve, and then, from her mother's house to her boyfriend Jason's parents' house ("me and my mom didn't get along for a while") and then back into the small house where her mother, who worked part-time as a bartender at the local country club, was living with a new man, a correctional officer at the penitentiary. Angel had dropped out of school two years before I met her, because the people there were "regular pains in the butt." She broke up with her boyfriend Jason and was dating someone else but then, after a night of reconnection, discovered she was pregnant. She was still in love with Jason, the father of her ten, month-old-son, Ben, even though their relationship was off and on, and sometimes violent.

Moving from Alabama had been hard. Schoolmates at the new town had made fun of her clothes and her accent, and she hadn't found many friends. She still spoke with longing of her friends and cousins back in Alabama.

As to her literacy life, she didn't remember anyone reading to her when she was little, though she remembered that there were lots of books in her grandma's trailer, and now she liked to read just about anything except westerns. Her favorite book was Shel Silverstein's *Where the Sidewalk Ends,* but she said,

> actually I'm a little slower, like I've been in learning classes, like special ed classes, almost my whole entire life so I'm behind schedule on my reading, but I used to have like hooked-on-phonics games and all that stuff because I was a little slower on reading. But I'm getting better, so I'm happy.

Chief among her activities now, in addition to caring for her son, taking two courses at the Alyssa Learning Center—spelling and personal development; she had just finished up an algebra class that, an administrator told me, was about at a seventh-grade level—and looking for work, was her involvement with a local group that supported teen mothers. This group gave teen mothers a chance to talk to other young moms, helped them learn new ways of playing with their children and encouraged them to serve on "parent panels" at local schools, speaking to students about the difficulties of being a teen parent. Being a teen mother seemed to have given Angel a kind of celebrity, a kind of authority among her peers, and an identity that she had sorely needed.

> **Angel:** Once I was at a school all by myself so I was kind of nervous. That was my third panel.
>
> **Cynthia:** And people ask you questions?
>
> **Angel:** About like, they ask about Jason, if we're still together, they ask about money . . . they ask about the most embarrassing thing, what people think of me. . . . It gets pretty detailish but we're allowed to pass, like if they're asking questions about sex and stuff, we're not allowed to answer because the panel is supposed to keep teens from getting pregnant.
>
> **Cynthia:** How does asking questions about sex—violate that?
>
> **Angel:** I guess if they ask like if we're still having sex, and we say we are . . . we're supposed to keep kids from having sex and getting pregnant. We tell 'em basically the bottom line is, wait, y' know, make sure that the person is the one you want to spend the rest of your life with. Every teen that I'm around, like my sister's age, they say, it's so cool, it's so cool, you got a baby, and I'm like un-uh. I am *not* cool because I have a baby. The baby is cool, but I'm not cool because I have a baby. . . .So we help them see how it is . . . It's really neat . . .

Shortly after her family had moved to Stonesville, Angel's father had been relocated to a prison in another state. Angel said,

> I think the last time I seen him I was like—nine. This year he sent me a Christmas card
> and a mother's day card. He writes me all the time but I take forever to write him back;
> I haven't written him in like—two months. He's supposed to get out next November.
> He says he's going to move to Stonesville just so he can be with me and Ben. I told him
> he's only got one more chance so if he messes up and ends up back in jail this time I'm
> not going to have anything to do with him.

Though she was a girl who had been in "learning classes" her "whole entire
life," Angel's relationship with her father had been entirely mediated through
reading and writing for almost nine years: Angel, a student who had always
been in lower-track classes, was very involved in a "literacy practice that the
school did not acknowledge" (Luttrell & Parker 2001, 243); it was a kind of
private reading and writing very different from that more public writing she
did, on worksheets at the Alyssa Learning Center.

In addition to that more private writing, and the reading of poetry, Angel
read the magazine *American Baby*, which probably helped her proclaim—and
learn information important to—her new and troubling and very important
identity as a teen mother (Finders 1997). "I get that magazine every month I
perscribe to it," Angel said.

Gabriel

"My baby's father is an extremely big loser"

Gabriel Banks was a girl with a purple streak running through her yellow
hair and silver glitter on her eyelids and cheeks; she wore velveteen sweatpants
in a wide array of soft pastel colors. When I asked her to describe herself
in one word, she replied quickly, "bitchy," and then corrected herself, "no,
impatient." She explained her unusual name by saying that her birth father's
name was Obadiah—"he's one of the books in the Old Testament—and my
mother wanted to keep it biblical." Edgy, flat of affect, casual, Gabriel quickly
made clear to me that she wasn't sure of the last name of the father of her baby,
that she wasn't particularly happy or particularly sad that she was pregnant,
and that she was sure she could afford to raise the baby alone, both "mentally"
and financially. "My mother will help me," she said, and, "I'm not a big fan of
abortion."

Though I'll describe conversations with other middle-class teen mothers
in later chapters, Gabriel was the only young woman of these four who

described herself as "upper middle class" ("my father's a systems analyst, he's quite well-off; my mother's manic depressive and schizophrenic; she has five credit cards and she goes on these shopping jags, which kind of screws up the finances sometimes"); she was also the only one who said she had been in "honors classes, but not AP classes, honors." She was the most competent and ambitious reader of the four young women I describe in this chapter; she was the only one who listed many books she had read or enjoyed reading: not only *A Clockwork Orange, Slaughterhouse Five,* and *The Experiment,* but many other science fiction and fantasy novels as well. She didn't particularly like English, she said, but she knew she was good at it.

I only met Gabriel a few times; the first time I met her I had brought with me the strange little children's book *Doll Baby* (2000) by Eve Bunting. It's a short book, and a peculiar one, and I thought it might contrast interestingly with the novels Casey, Angel, and I were exploring. When neither Casey nor Angel showed up that day, Melinda introduced me to Gabriel, who immediately began telling me what I thought of as very personal information about herself. ("The father of my baby is an extremely big loser. He's a whole lot older than me. I would never tell him I was pregnant" and "I began cutting myself when I was twelve till I was like fourteen. It was like the physical pain helped me feel better about the emotional pain. And I saw other girls doing it there so that's how I got the idea. And I came to the understanding when I was like thirteen that I would probably get pregnant young. So I wasn't shocked when I found out I was pregnant, I expected it.") For privacy, we moved into a little nurse's office; there I learned more about her reading habits, her family relationships, and her perspectives on being an unwed pregnant girl:

> Generally media portrays it's the girls fault if she gets pregnant. Now, I think that's wrong. Okay this sounds bad but if two girls had sex they wouldn't have a baby—it's both people's fault. I know this is a big issue but I think they should make condoms available at school in a little basket or in the nurses' office because a lot of guys are extremely shy to go to the drug store or something . . .

She said, "I sort of figure I'll be happy when the baby comes."

After we'd talked a while we read *Doll Baby* together. This is a picture book about avoiding unwed pregnancy, written for nine-year-olds. Gabriel said she felt "pity" for the girl in the story, who gets pregnant, and whose boyfriend leaves her. Gabriel said she thought the story seemed fairly true to life:

> **Gabriel:** If the boyfriend told the story instead of the girl, he'd say he had a girlfriend and yes they had sex but no way was it his child. I guess later he got sent away, and

then even later came back and didn't think about the girl.

Cynthia: Why do you think the girl in the story has a stepfather? (This was a leading question; I was hoping she'd notice the stereotypical broken family the pregnant girl in the story belongs to.)

Gabriel: 'Cause people don't generally stay together these days.

Later, Gabriel sat looking at the book in her lap. "The lady who wrote this would probably think I'm a slut," she said. And then, looking up, "Half of it is crap anyways. That whole idea that teens sexually act out because they're angry at whoever so they get pregnant so they have an excuse to not live at home, that's crap."

She turned the pink-and-blue pages of *Doll Baby* quietly for a while, looking over her three-months-pregnant belly. "This girl doesn't know what she's getting herself into," she said.

Casey

"I learned at an early age what a pap smear was"

When I met Casey Howard I remembered Lisa Dodson's description of how different the lives of poor women are from what we imagine girls experience; she writes that in our culture we perpetuate "the fantasy of soft girlishness against the truth of hard female lives" (Dodson 1998, 187). Serene behind her round glasses, with her straight brown hair pulled back into a neat ponytail, Casey Howard seemed older than her nineteen years.

As I talked with Casey it occurred to me that she had been interviewed many times before, that she was familiar with this way of presenting herself—more familiar with this whole process, possibly, than I was—and that she often hoped to shock me. She had that composure that Adam Phillips (1993) calls "self-holding and self-hiding" (46), that composure that is "like a dare," challenging the "idea of accurate recognition" (46). Casey had a habit of ending her sentences with the word "so," a self-conscious period, a somewhat defensive marker, that seemed to challenge me, the awkward, middle-aged interviewer. Melinda, who sat quietly at the front desk in the career room at the Alyssa Learning Center, typing information into her computer and occasionally interviewing students, had set up my meeting with Casey. Melinda said that Casey stopped by the center often after she heard of my interest in interviewing her, asking, is that woman who wants to read with young mothers coming by?

I felt a little bit wanted, then, by this young woman, and I appreciated being wanted. I began to see her, this newly married mother of a three-month-old, as a mix of maturity and immaturity, determination, confidence, and confusion.

I met and spoke with Casey throughout the spring and summer semesters of 2003. Using tape recordings, hand-written notes, and her own written materials, I began to parse Casey's story. To interpret her story, I used strategies for life-narrative analysis suggested by Stanton Wortham (2001) in *Narratives in Action: A Strategy for Research and Analysis* and by Elinor Ochs and Lisa Capps (2001) in *Living Narrative: Creating Lives in Everyday Storytelling*. Wortham argues that the self can be transformed through the relationship between the story the narrator is telling and her positioning of self within that autobiographical narrative; Ochs and Capps focus on personal narratives that are co-constructed and on the moral stances speakers build through these conversations.

I hope to describe in these pages the emotional significance of reading in Casey's life. When I write of the emotional significance of reading I hearken back to Robert Solomon's (1986) seminal essay, "Literacy and the Education of the Emotions," in which he argues that one purpose of literature is to "educate the emotions," which he defines as providing the reader with "an opportunity to have an emotion, to learn when it is appropriate and when inappropriate, to learn its vicissitudes and, if the term isn't too jarring, its logic" (45). Through reading, Casey worked out and thought through difficult emotions and perhaps began to see herself in new ways. I hope to show how reading, talking about that reading, and—as Wortham suggests—telling her life story were transformative for her.

In our earliest meeting Casey had presented herself—with some strain, I thought—as a woman whose life was much more than fine. She lived in a "really cute" duplex with her husband, Sam, who had a good job at a local home improvement store. He was twenty-six—quite a bit older than Casey—and she had planned out her relationship to him carefully. Prior to meeting him, she had moved out of her mother's house, dropped out of high school, and had been working at a local inn: she proudly explained that she had worked her way up from maid to manager in less than a year. When she "started hearing about this guy, Sam," she quit her job at the inn and found another one, working as an employee of Sam's. "It was risky, I know, but he sounded just right for me," she said, and she'd quickly broken off another relationship ("I gave that boyfriend a eighth of pot as a going-away present") and started going out with Sam. Her mother, from whom she had been estranged for some years, felt better about

Casey's life now, and they were all friends. Her mother liked Sam "because she knows that when he gets angry, he just gets real quiet. And he doesn't do drugs."

They had married in October; Casey's son, Russell, was born two months later. Casey and her husband Sam worked hard at their marriage, which for many reasons, was strained: the difference in their ages, her problems with anger management, money problems, and the stress of having a new baby. Casey's typical day centered on caring for her baby—feeding him, putting him "down for a nap"—and helping her mother, who had recently begun treatment for breast cancer, and ran a daycare center out of her home.

Casey felt fairly confident about raising her son, she said, and she was proud to have married into Sam's family, in which everybody was college-educated. ("Even Sam has two years of college.") She said that since she had her son she had become more motivated to finish high school, particularly because Sam wanted her to, and that she wanted to go on to college and become an art therapist. According to school records, she had not yet completed tenth grade; during the semesters I worked with her she did not take any classes at the Alyssa Learning Center. But at our first meeting she said she felt that overall her life was "pretty fun." Especially, "over the last year. I mean, I'm back together with my mom, and I met Sam, and I had Russ! So."

In our second conversation Casey told me that, at her mother's daycare center, she had been reading *Thomas the Tank Engine* books to the children and, to a "really smart" four-year-old, *Harry Potter and the Sorcerer's Stone*, which she found "kind of hard." I asked Casey if she had started reading more or less since her son was born.

Casey: Well, actually, when I was pregnant I never read. 'Cause it was so hard for me. And my husband got me reading every night. We read—we read books about pregnancy and stuff like that. He got me reading every night, and I had to read out loud to him and that has helped a little bit. So it became our routine that we read every night. We love it.

Cynthia: Are you still reading? What kinds of things are you reading now?

Casey: I don't know. What are we reading? We have a lot of—a lot of books. History books is what we like to read. I mean—just—he has a bunch of—just tons of books and we'll pick out books here and there and just—Russ likes to look at the pictures and to listen to us. Hear us read.

Cynthia: What about at home when you were growing up?

Casey: Well, let's see. When I was five I was in foster care, so. Didn't have much home-life there.

Cynthia: And why were you in foster care?

Casey: Um that was—during my mom and my biological father's custody battle between—for me and Joe, my brother. And there was abuse and they thought my mom was doing it and my dad was really doing it. So. It was hard because my mom had boyfriends, and she married Bill and that wasn't good. I didn't like him, and I was forced to call him dad. You know.

Casey spoke, as we all always do, into and against and because of larger societal conversations (Wortham 2001). In this particular case, Casey spoke into a conversation about the kind of girl who gets pregnant young, about the value of reading, and about what family relationships should look like.

In this brief bit of conversation Casey repeated three times the phrase "reading every night," and she repeated that her husband has "a lot of books," "just tons of books." I suspect that in this early conversation with me, she was presenting herself as a good student and trying to impress me with the idea that, as a young wife and mother, she is working hard as well to learn to read better than she does. She's annoyed when I ask for specifics: It doesn't really matter to her what the books she reads are about, just that there were a lot of them, and they are associated with her husband Sam, a man she is alternately proud of ("my husband") and affectionately, self-consciously teasing of ("the dork"). She believes that it had "helped a little bit" for her to read out loud every night to her husband, and she assumes that her husband's reading is an individual achievement that he should be proud of (Cherland 1994). When Casey says later that Sam "reads mythology books and stuff like that. He reads all the time. He's very intelligent" she suggests that she believes, as Cherland (1994) suggests some students do, that "being a reader means being smart" (88).

It is important also to Casey that her husband read *books*, not articles or magazines. This is a somewhat old-fashioned definition of literacy: Casey doesn't mention her husband reading the sports page or the police blotter; he doesn't analyze movie images or read blogs online; it seems clear that for Casey in reading literature one acquires what Anyon (1981) calls a kind of "'prestigious knowledge' (as cited in Cherland 1994, 121)—the kind of knowledge . . . associated with the advantages of the upper classes, and . . . viewed as a kind of 'cultural capital' that would be valuable later in life" (Cherland 1994, 121). Cherland (1994) writes that she suspects people who assume, as Casey seems to, and most probably have been taught to think in school, that literary knowledge consists mostly of facts and dates and literary terms, and who think this kind of knowledge can be traded for good grades, college degrees, and good jobs, are sadly mistaken. Cherland (1994) suggests that "what counts as knowledge" (123), as it is organized by schools, is different for working-class students like Casey than it is for children of the wealthy (123). I find it poignant, then, when Casey mentions that her son Russ likes to hear his parents read aloud to each other; I think that Casey hopes that by letting him listen to her read she's providing her son with advantages she didn't have, I think she's hoping that this background will help him move up more securely into the middle class. This is one reason also, as she mentions later, that she has three-month-old Russ listen to a Mozart CD every night before he goes to sleep. ("He listens to classical music because it helps develop his brain.")

Abuse and Learning to Read

When she briefly mentions her mother forcing her to call her stepfather Bill "Dad," Casey uses the expression "you know" in a way that is very powerful. Implicit in that "you know" is an entire story, one Casey suggests that we both know pretty well, of the mother trying to force a good relationship between the stepfather and the stepchild, attempting to create a relationship through naming. Casey tells this to me as if we both know that this will never work; she tells this to me in a way that is meant to bond us together as two women more psychologically sophisticated than her mother, who, in Casey's stories, occupies multiple roles and is presented as victim, brave cancer survivor, confused wife, economic help, close friend, enemy, and hard-nosed entrepreneur.

> **Casey:** And then once they got divorced—that was in '92 and then she married Alex. And I extremely hated him, I hated him so much, but then they got married and had my little sister Nancy, and, you know. Alex tried to raise me right. It's tough love, he'd always tell me, it's just tough love. And I'm like, okay, whatever (laughing). But you know and then you know our relationship, I started calling him dad. I love him so much. And then, my son has his middle name. My son's middle name is the same as my dad's middle name. James.
>
> **Cynthia:** And he was your mom's—second?
>
> **Casey:** Third. (Big sigh). Third husband, yeah.
>
> **Cynthia:** So he—
>
> **Casey:** Growing up wasn't fun. I mean, I had my brother, and that was about it.
>
> **Cynthia:** So there wasn't much reading going on.

Casey: Bill taught me to read. And he taught me—what was it—is your mom a—dealing with a llama. And he taught me to read that book and I think I read that book a million times. And—Doctor Seuss books is what we had. But I don't remember many books.

Cynthia: And was that a good time, with Bill?

Casey: That was the only good time with Bill.

Cynthia: That could have been scary too.

Casey: No. He was a different person during the day than he was at night.

Cynthia: So you have good memories of reading? What about in school?

Casey: I never paid attention in school. I didn't like to read and I didn't like to do the work.

Cynthia: Can you remember any books you read in school that you liked?

Casey: No.

It became clear through our conversations that Casey had been taught to read, when she was seven, by her first stepfather, Bill, a high school baseball coach, whom she later saw throw her little sister against the wall, and who abused her sexually when her mother was asleep. She felt Bill wasn't that different from her biological father. As Casey said,

> when I was in foster care when I was five, I'd go visit my biological father, and after every visit I went straight to Saint Mary's Hospital, straight to Saint Mary's . . . I learned at an early age what a pap smear was. And it was beyond horrible and then after the custody battle I went back to live with my mom and she got in a relationship with Bill and he did those things, too.

In *Too Scared to Learn: Women, Violence, and Education*, Dr. Jenny Horsman (2000), a community-based literacy theorist, educator, and researcher, describes the ways in which talk about domestic violence and sexual abuse is silenced in adult literacy programs. Horsman suggests that "literacy workers" are more open to talking with their students about the "bad school experiences . . . which are seen as the reason that children fall through the cracks and fail to learn" than they are to talking about violence and family sexual abuse (55). Horsman writes that "we do not talk about the ways in which focusing on learning to read can remind a woman of when she was a child trying to learn and that the connection to childhood may be terrifying"(55). Horsman suggests that violence against women is a common and commonly accepted attribute of our culture, and that teachers in community colleges or adult education programs are working with people who have been subject to violence more often than they realize.

During the rest of the conversation recorded above, Casey talks about Alex, her second stepfather, remembering hating him. Casey enacts her emotional travels with him as she describes this hatred, then mocks him lovingly when she says he tried to raise her "right." She smiles wide when she repeats his words that his attempts to discipline her were "tough love, just tough love"; she laughs as she remembers how rebellious she was and imitates the flippant language of her younger self ("I'm like, whatever"). In this "authoring" (Wortham 2001), Casey speaks in three voices: the exasperated voice of her stepfather, the voice of a community that has ideas about what it means to raise a young woman "right," and the voice of her younger self. It's good to see that she can feel affection for that old rebellious self and that she can remember and appreciate, from her new vantage point of mother, her stepfather's attempts to parent her well. She speaks, as she often does in her conversations with me, to the whole question of what it means to be a good parent. Certainly a good father teaches his daughter (or stepdaughter) to read (Brandt, 2001). A good father also shows "tough love" to his cursing, drug-taking, late-night-partying stepdaughter. (Says Casey, with some pride: "I was not a good teen. No.")

And in Casey's story about her stepfather Alex, we see the power of naming. Casey finally is not forced to call anyone her father, but can act with some agency, and, given that freedom and a man who seems not to abuse her, chooses at last to call this man dad. "I love him so much," she says of this third father figure; she loves him so much that she gives her baby son his middle name. At the time Casey told me this story, this last stepfather Alex, this good stepfather, (with whom, Casey said, "there's no violence, I mean he hit [my mother] once, 6–7 years ago, and that was it") was not living with her mother any longer.

Trauma and the Transformative Power of Reading

During one of the conversations Casey and I shared, Angel Brown breezed into the room. She protested that she was not "majorly late" for our meeting and told us that her old car had broken down again. This was the first time she and Casey had met; they introduced themselves to each other primarily by comparing their experiences of pregnancy.

(**Casey:** "I was big and fat for my wedding, I was like 4–6 months pregnant." **Angel:** I didn't do—whaddayacallit—Lamaze. I watched TV. I watched the pregnancy channel." **Cynthia:** "The pregnancy channel?" **Casey:** "TLC. A Baby's Story and Maternity Ward." **Angel:** "Yeah, and Delivery Room.")

I suspect that Casey felt a little put out that Angel entered into our conversation, because she made sure that my attention returned to her by telling me that one of her favorite books was something like "A Boy That Was Lost, or A Boy Called It."

> **Cynthia:** *A Child Called It* by Dave Pelzer?
>
> **Casey:** Yeah. I connected so well with that book.
>
> **Cynthia:** Dave Pelzer's book?
>
> **Casey:** Yeah.
>
> **Cynthia:** Because I know there's some question about whether it's true or not.
>
> **Casey:** Really?
>
> **Cynthia:** It's a biography, right, an autobiography?
>
> **Casey:** Yeah. His childhood and what he went through . . . I mean, his mother was cruel, beyond cruel to him. She was horrible. And I connected so well with that because it's my past, and it made sense. And it related to so many things for me.

A Child Called It (1995), an autobiography subtitled *One Child's Courage to Survive*, is a story of child abuse that was published in 1995 and has been on *The New York Times* and *USA Today* best-seller lists. Categorized as "self-help/psychology/inspiration" the book concerns the childhood of the main character, the young Dave Pelzer, who is systematically starved; made to eat feces, ammonia, dishwashing soap, and dirt; called "a little shit," "the Boy," and "It"; made to sleep on an army cot in the basement away from the rest of the family; and in one instance forced to wave his hand over the fire on a stove. His mother—who commits all this abuse—also breaks his arm, stabs him in the stomach, and forces him to run alongside the car when she drives his brothers to school. Articles that describe the story behind the book call Dave Pelzer's the third-worst case of child abuse in California state history.

In *A Child Called It*, Pelzer's mother, Catherine Rovea, is presented as an evil, monstrous, out-of-control woman. There is no suggestion of any motivation for her actions; she changes—from one chapter to the next, suddenly, when Dave enters second grade—from a loving, nurturing, imaginative, cheerful, well-dressed and carefully made-up woman into an overweight, alcoholic, unkempt sadist. This mother "sneers," "snarls," "snaps," "screams," and occasionally slumps over when "the booze (had) her in a deep six" (Pelzer 1995, 74). There is very little moral ambiguity in the story, no sense of the history of the marriage between the character Dave's parents, no sense of his grandparents' history. In fact, I learned more about the facts of his parents' life from reading a brief article about the book than I did from reading the book. Though the story is set in the 1950s, when laws were not in place requiring teachers to report cases of child abuse, some readers have suggested that the story is too bad to be true: it's not until Dave is in the fifth grade that a kindly teacher notices that the child wears rags, has bruises all over his body, and never brings lunch to school.

The book is published by the same company that puts out the *Chicken Soup for the Soul* books: it's of the inspirational best-seller genre; on the cover of the copy I read is a drawing of a hand coming out of the clouds, gently raising the chin of a young white boy—Dave, one assumes. Though I had found this book badly written and sensational, aiming baldly to shock, reading it had been important to Casey in many ways.

> **Cynthia:** Talk more about what the book did for you.
>
> **Casey:** Made me see I wasn't the only one out there—that had this—in their life. That there's people that do understand. What's his name?
>
> **Cynthia:** Dave Pelzer. I think. P-E-L-Z-E-R. One's called something like "lost boy."
>
> **Angel:** You can look in the library.
>
> **Casey:** I mean I just connected so well with it and it's like—you knew what he was feeling. Cause I've felt that, and just to know there's other people out there, that have felt that.
>
> **Cynthia:** And—and—what does he—how does it end?
>
> **Casey:** Well it goes on to the next book that I haven't read yet, so. I think he was— lonely and went to a foster home for a while? I don't remember how it ended. But I've read it so many times.

Here, Casey describes reading as having been lifesaving for her, "just to know that there's other people out there, that have felt that way." Learning, through reading this book, that others had experiences like—perhaps worse than—her own helped her feel less alone as she tried to make sense of her fragmented memories. In her language, there is the diction of therapy—"I just connected so well with it." The phrase has the whiff of the couch, not surprising from a young woman who has been in and out of treatment centers for much of her adolescence. In this conversation, Casey is performing for me, trying to shock me perhaps, certainly ensuring that she's got my attention. It's also clear, though, that the experiences she describes are central to her sense of who she is.

Cynthia: It (*A Child Called It*) meant a lot to you. What was going on in your life then?

Casey: Well, my stepdad Alex. I call him my dad now. He always told me he didn't want anybody to force me to talk about what happened. In my past. Until I was ready. Well, I was trying to get ready to talk about it. Put two and two together and figure out what happened. 'Cause I don't remember. 'Cause as a young child you block that stuff out of your brain, your brain blocks it out. I tried to figure out what happened cause I don't remember. So I was—I found that book and it really helped me start talking about things.

Cynthia: Helped you think about it?

Casey: Sure.

Cynthia: Helped you put it together.

Casey: And it helped my stepdad too. He had problems with his biological father too, with abuse and stuff, so it was easier to talk to him because he understood.

In *Living Narrative*, their book about the everyday conversations that make up our lives, Elinor Ochs and Lisa Capps (2001) discuss the complexity of memory. They explain that present experience affects the ways in which we remember the past and that much of what we remember is affected by the stereotypes of our culture. They also discuss some of the ways that trauma affects memory.

The experiences of sexual abuse Casey suffered were for some time inaccessible to her explicit memory, unavailable for narration, not "tellable" (Ochs & Capps 2001, 171). Many survivors of trauma have what Ochs and Capps call "profound narrative fragmentation"; they are "plagued by flashes of remembered sights, sounds, smells, and other sensations (and) struggle to articulate distressing events"(171). Even though their minds are "overwhelmed," as Casey's was, by the trauma of child sexual abuse that "defeats our capacity to organize it," even though this experience may not be accessible to language, at the same time, the body is aware of what happened, keeping score, showing symptoms like "numbing," nightmares, or avoidance (171).

Ochs and Capps describe how being able to tell your story, to knit thoughts and actions together, is a profound part of psychological well-being. They write of how "cultural plot lines" can be healing (221), allowing tellers to make sense of traumatic or damaging events by placing them into familiar, widely accepted story templates. Though there is usually some tension between the need to render your experiences specifically and personally and the need to understand those experiences in a manner that is culturally familiar and acceptable to others, placing your specific life story into such a template can be "potentially comforting" (221) as, I would argue, placing her half-remembered traumatic experiences into the template provided by the story of *A Child Called It* was comforting to Casey.

A Child Called It has that "simple syntax, elementary realism, repetitive vocabulary, and authorial interpretation" that Janice Radway (1984) writes of when she describes romance novels, those elements that "together create a verbal structure that can be decoded easily and quickly on the basis of previously mastered cultural codes and conventions" (197). And, like the romance readers Radway describes, Casey read *A Child Called It* "so many times": "If this phenomenon of repetitive reading is accorded the importance it deserves, it becomes clear that . . . novels function for their reader, on one level at least, as the ritualistic repetition of a single, immutable cultural myth" (198). *A Child Called It* may have worked as a cultural myth into which Casey placed her fragmented and frightening experiences each time she read it. This placing of her own story onto the written story of *A Child Called It* may have helped Casey structure her experiences in a new way.

The healing aspects of reading *A Child Called It* over and over again would be complicated, slow, and at best partial, however. Ochs and Capps write that "the plotting of psychic interiors on to comforting narrative frames is full of obstacles, not the least of which is the nagging sensation that one's life is more fragmented than the experiential world depicted in cultural stories" (221). One example of the ways in which Casey's experience is more fragmented than the story in *A Child Called It* is that Casey was abused by two people—a parent and a stepparent—rather than one; another difference between Casey's story and Dave's is gender.

As an abused young woman reading *A Child Called It*, Casey identified with the abused young man in the story; feminist theorist Judith Fetterly might say that she was "identifying against herself" (quoted in Blackford 2004, 17). "In this historical context," writes Cherland (1994), also citing Fetterley, "it should not be surprising that the female reader of this male-authored and male-identified literary canon is required, when she reads, to identify herself as male and thus to identify against herself, in order to share in the meaning of the work" (14). It may be that Casey identifies herself as male as she reads Pelzer's autobiography; she may also find herself "implicated in the representation of the female character"—in this case, the abusive mother (Blackford 2004, 17).

In the conversational segment about reading with her stepfather, above, Casey describes a somewhat younger, more vulnerable self. As she retells this story she "enacts" the younger self as she talks about this younger self's experiences (Wortham 2001). Her sentences become shorter ("In my past. Until I was ready."), her voice a little softer. When she says, "And it helped my stepdad too, he had problems with his biological father too with abuse and stuff, so it was easier to talk to him because he understood," she's aligning herself with an adult caretaker who himself was wounded by abuse, but who showed her, perhaps for the first time, how a caring father might behave. This stepfather, giving her the privacy and the agency to make decisions in her own time and reading with her this book that helped them both begin to think and talk about past experiences of abuse, seems to have begun to help Casey feel safe enough to remember and think and even talk about her experiences. As she told me this memory of conversations and reading with her stepfather, Casey moved from a vulnerable child to a compassionate adult, expressing care for her stepfather, and thereby enacting a stronger self. In *Narratives in Action*, Wortham describes how it is in the interaction between the representation of self and the enactment of that representation that the self is transformed. As with the repetitious reading of *A Child Called It*, this parallel description and performance of a strong and less vulnerable self would have to happen many times in order to bring about a more than partial healing. And yet in these conversations with me, and in Casey's reading, that healing, that transformation, has begun.

"I'm not one of these that'd leave my baby in a trash can"

Casey: And like—I was—as I was growing up—I always overheard, you're going to eventually abuse your kid, 'cause you were abused. And I worry about anger. Because I'm on medication to control my anger and I have a real bad anger issue and there are times when Sam is at work, I just take Russell to my mom's. Because I'm just, I'm never at my house unless Sam is there. I'm too scared to be alone with him, so.

Cynthia: But you're doing a good job!

Casey: Yeah, yeah, but my biggest fear is, you know, and then I was watching *Crossing Jordan* [a television show] last week and the one baby, the one mother had the water too high and she scalded the baby, and there was a baby up towards I think it was Waterford. My friend Eliza, she goes around to schools and she talks about pregnant—

Angel: Parent panel. She's one of those I do my parent panels with.

Casey: Eliza?

Angel: Um-hm.

Casey: Really. She's so cool, I love her to death.

Angel: She's got short blond hair? Brownish blonde?

Casey: Yeah, and she's got a little boy named Dustin.

Angel: Uh-hum.

Casey: Yup, Dustin's my buddy.

Angel: We got a parent panel—ummm—end of the month. Up in Hatfield.

Casey: I didn't know she did that. But she's—she's so (inaudible). But there was a—one of the babies—died. The parents she was working with. They suspected abuse. A few days later well the police went over there and checked it out, well, DFS went over there and apparently the baby died.

Angel: Towards Waterford?

Casey: I think it was. And then well they were saying they've (inaudible). But they thought it was abuse. Because he was sucking candy. So that—

Angel: Was it somebody she was babysitting for?

Casey: She does—the program that she's in I guess. One of the parents, the couples, their baby died.

Angel: I didn't know she did that.

Casey: Eliza Curtis.

Angel's interruption of Casey's talk is borne partly of Angel's extreme pride about the parent panels she's involved in. Also, she's just trying to get back into the conversation. The stories these two girls tell each other are very familiar to me: Many of the teen moms I spoke with told stories of mothers who had abused or neglected or killed their children; these narratives seemed to be an important part of these young women's "figured world." Casey and Angel use the stories they tell about other mothers as Holland and her co-authors (1998, 71) describe, as "a cultural vehicle for identity formation." In telling these stories, the girls say to each other, and to outsiders, "We're all part of the same figured world, we're all teen moms; we know about this."

In some ways, these stories also had a moral purpose: They were markers against which the young women compared themselves: "I'm not one of these that'd leave my baby in a trash can," Brenda said. Angel told of younger women whom she met through her parent panels who hit their children or did not feed them well. Casey and Angel both made references to a local teenager who had been arrested for abandoning her baby, a story that was much in the news. Often in the telling of these stories, the girls expressed scorn for the women and thus cast themselves as virtuous, a common habit in tellers of stories, Ochs and Capps (2001, 137) tell us.

The stories about other young women who abuse their children, like the one Casey tells Angel in conversational segment above, are certainly also expressions of anxiety. See how Casey scares Angel with her story, and see how the fact that this investigation into parental abuse might have happened to a parent Angel knows, and in a town close to hers, makes her fear more intense. These stories fascinate in their shock; they create a picture that combines what psychoanalyst Jessica Benjamin (1988) calls "the present desolate condition of motherhood" and "the hardness and profligacy of the culture" (214). They also preserve the image of the bad, all-powerful, evil mother whom we see in *A Child Called It*. In that these young mothers' stories do this, there may be evidence of what Benjamin calls "splitting": an inability to integrate hate with love, failure with success, the good parts of the mother-self with the weak parts: "this failure of integration is the essential element in splitting" (Benjamin 1988, 211).

Finally, the stories these young women told also speak of their fantasies and fears of abuse. In Casey's poignant explanation of the reason she takes her son to her mother's every day—her knowledge that the abused often becomes the abuser—I see an example of moral thinking. Through raising her son, Russ, Casey was learning that "mother-love" is really a mix of emotions—sorrow, tenderness, impatience, a sense of duty, affection, anger, and perhaps despair. Sara Ruddick might say that, when Casey took her son to her mother's every day in order to protect him from her problems with "anger management," she was learning how to enact the virtue of commitment to her child's safety (Ruddick 1989, 67).

Casey is then, in some ways, because of her experiences of abuse and because of the emotional wisdom she is gaining through her young motherhood, much older emotionally than other students her age might be. Thus, when Casey reads *A Child Called It*, the book may miss its mark: Though Casey is immature in some ways (her need to tell me stories about her friends who are in jail points up a desire to shock, which suggests immaturity), Casey's moral learning—as she works through her feelings for her son, as she helps her mother at the daycare center, as she wrestles to keep communication open in her new marriage—is beginning to be much more complex, much more nuanced and mature than is the moral expression of the writers of the books she is ready—is *able*—to read. She is most probably aware in her life of moral issues that are less starkly framed than those in *A Child Called It*.

Elizabeth Ellsworth writes that this is often the case: there is often a mismatch between "who a curriculum thinks its students are or should be" and who those students really are. Ellsworth (1997) wonders, in her book *Teaching Positions: Difference, Pedagogy, and the Power of Address*, about how that mismatch ("the fact that all modes of address miss their audience in some way or other") can be turned into a resource for teachers (38). Ellsworth tells us that one space the mismatch between student and curriculum opens up is the space of audience: in part, the power of *A Child Called It*, for Casey, may have been in who the book thought its reader was; sensing herself as an audience with an identity different from the one she usually had when reading may have opened up a new imaginative space for Casey. The power of this book may have resided in its difference from other books Casey had read—the difference between what Casey had experienced as possible to say about a parent and what Pelzer actually says (Ellsworth 1997, 40). Or this book may have offered Casey a kind of freedom simply in that it opened up as possible to talk about an as-yet-secret topic. Finally, it may not have been the book that was helpful to Casey, really, at all, but rather the fact that her stepfather Alex took time to read and think and talk about this subject with her. After all, as Deborah Britzman (2006) tells us, it isn't even really the teacher who educates; "what educates is not the person but an emotional experience of relating that becomes the basis for further meaning" (166). This "emotional experience of relating" may be a large part of the education many teen mothers—and many abused young women—most need.

Conclusions

Bakhtin wrote that "the ideological becoming of a human being . . . is the process of selectively assimilating the words of others" (as quoted in Wortham, 2001, 147). Wortham comments on Bakhtin's statement by writing "This puts the Western self in an ironic position: struggling to articulate its own individual voice but able to do so only by speaking through others." I wondered, and I wonder still, how the words that Casey had assimilated helped and hindered her as she tried to become the multilayered, conscientious and forgetful, touchy and teasing, angry and tender, competitive and frightened, needy and independent self that I saw. In the classic text *Young, Poor, and Pregnant: The Psychology of Teenage Motherhood*, Musick (1993) has written that the findings of her research on the connection between abuse and early motherhood "tend to validate the clinical perceptions that for a sizable group of adolescent mothers, contemporary social and sexual relationships with males may be reenactments of patterns established earlier in life: lessons of victimization learned all too well" (91). In these pages we'll meet a few of the many young mothers who were not abused as children; still, I wonder how loudly the words of Casey's abusive father and stepfather ring in her ears as she tries to forge a new relationship with Sam, and I wonder as well, with Musick, about the manipulation and power struggles that might make up the "psychological context" of Casey's relationship with Sam, the context into which her son, Russell, was conceived (91).

"Years later, the wounds [of abuse] are still there," Musick writes (91). Casey told me she couldn't understand why her mother always picked abusive men to marry. ("She married at sixteen, maybe that's what screwed her up. And then she kinda stayed on that train because she thought that was all she could get.") She couldn't understand, either, how she had found a good man who didn't drink, do drugs, or commit abusive acts. Maybe the love of her mother and brother and of a stepfather who listened to her had something to do with her healing. Maybe finding a book about abuse, recognizing her own experiences in it, and reading that book over and over again had something to do with it as well.

On my last visit with her, Casey told me that she and Sam had gone to see her biological father one last time, and had introduced him to her baby, Russ. "Sam sat out in the car when I went to see him. He wouldn't let me go alone," she said. "My biological father's not in prison, but he deserves to be." After the visit she and Sam decided that "when Russ is old enough, we're gonna tell him his grandpa's dead. Because he might as well be."

In that last conversation, Casey also told me that reading would never be easy for her. Even when she read out loud, with her husband and her baby at her side, she said, "it's work, and it'll always be work for me." She admitted to being proud of herself, her husband, her baby, and her new life, though. She said with a laugh, "I'm still here. Sometimes it's hard to believe, after all I've been through, that I'm nineteen, I made it this far, and I'm still here."

Utah, 1979:
Two Months a Teacher

September 10, 1979—Letter to mom

My life is in smithereens! My third week of classes. In child development, I gave a lesson on self-esteem, where I explained that sometimes as we go through the day we feel people are taking bites out of us. Like this, I said, and bit an apple I'd brought in just for this purpose. I'd read it in a book somewhere, some professor suggested it. But the girls laughed! They all laughed at me! In my next class, English, a girl sauntered in and asked, "You gonna bite an apple for us?" A teacher from another school picked me up as I was walking forlornly home. I told her this story and she said, listen, you learn from your mistakes. So go ahead and make mistakes!!! *I'm doing it . . .*

I need to act more professional!!!! I wrote in my diary. The only problem was, I didn't know what it meant to be a professional teacher—were teachers professionals?—especially in this crazy school. One day, another teacher, the determined, hard-driving Liz Rosenstein (now principal of a high school in that same city) talked to me about professionalism and emotion: It's your job to keep pushing at the girls, being friendly, she said. The crazier and more outgoing you are, the more your classes will work. If a girl doesn't respond, that might hurt your feelings, but know that you have to keep going because this is your profession.

A professor from my graduate school program came to watch me teach. He noticed the way I interacted with a tall black student named Dainty. He'd said I sounded "teacherly" and "harsh" with her. I should watch myself more when I talk to students, he told me, treat them as I would treat their parents. Later, Liz said, "I wonder how classes are affected by the *teacher's* self-esteem."

September 27—Letter to mom

Liz Rosenstein says to make sure I don't waste the girls' time in class doing things they could do on their own. So I'm going to think up activities, expect nothing, and GO FOR IT. My child development class went well today even though I was totally unprepared—having expected to give a film, finding we didn't have the right projector, having expected Ginelle to teach the class, finding out that not only does her baby—what's his name? Krishna?—have an earache but her mother smashed the car, Ginelle got glass in her eyes, and she'll be out of school for weeks. Even though that was a mess, things are going better because I shoved the tables together and am sitting with the girls instead of at my desk. Still, I tend to be baffled and overwrought, vacillating between this teacher role and this other as-yet-undefined-facilitator-friend-person-role—the role they say you're supposed to have in alternative schools. I realize I'm vulnerable because my life in this school matters more to me than it does to my students—I'm more invested—this classroom is my whole professional future, the girls have other lives, they're just passing through.

In classes, conversations kept veering off course. In English, we talked about the difficulty of communication, and in consumer ed, about what it's like when your water breaks, and about Geri Wilson, who didn't know she was pregnant until she was in labor. Out in the hall I overheard Dainty saying I was "the sorriest teacher," and in foods class, Deb Espinoza, holding one-month-old Moses against her shoulder, patting him on the back, asked me, "Cindy, am I flunking any of your classes yet?"

I had dreams full of babies and dreams full of classes in which all my students loved me. One student asked if I'd ever smoked pot—should she even be allowed to ask me questions like that? Another, eight months pregnant, tottered in during lunch, spread a baby blanket over a table and began eating a peanut butter sandwich. As she ate, she talked about how lonely she was, having just left her mother for the first time, having just moved to this state with her husband from Georgia. A student in child development asked me what to do about her husband: He didn't like holding the baby because he was afraid the baby would poop on him. I wrote in my diary: *I may be overwhelmed, I may be confused, but I sure am working hard.*

I took the advice of the minister's wife who taught down the hall and called Utah High School and had them send over some unused textbooks. I felt like I was copping out by using them—I had wanted to do more imaginative things in my classes—but having the textbooks did make my English class more organized. We read "The Necklace" and "Young Goodman Brown" out loud and I taught the girls vocabulary words like "cherish," "blunder," and "nimble." I began to feel—and I thought the girls began to feel—as if I was doing my job as I was supposed to.

October 20—Letter to mom

In gym every morning, mom, I watch ten big-tummied pregnant girls trying to hoist the volleyball net—a funny sight. I'm getting better at volleyball but I don't know if I'm getting better at teaching. Dainty came to visit me at lunch today. She's tall, older than the other girls, a mother already. She has a part-time job and sometimes wears suits and high heels to school.

She plays a mean game of volleyball.

*   "I tell you, Cindy," she said, "You got to do better than this. You just don't be usin' your head. These girls are pregnant, they've got things to think about, they ain't gonna do that homework you keep givin' them. And in English, that Hawthorne, what kinda shit is that? Most boring stuff I've ever read."*

*   I just have to learn more, work harder, I know.*

Two months a teacher.

Chapter 4

The Teen Moms' Book Club

Beginnings

When, just before Christmas 2003, I drove into the little downtown of Alyssa, to the learning center where I hoped to start the Teen Moms' Book Club, I thought back on the confusion and wonder I'd felt when I first taught young mothers at the Teen Moms' Program years earlier. Thinking about my students at the Teen Moms' Program, in 2002, I had read twenty-five young-adult novels about pregnant and mothering teens, wondering how teachers might be able to use those books, speculating that the books might serve as a kind of "community-through-literature" for pregnant and mothering teens (Coffel 2002, 19). Now I was going to find out if my ideas made sense. I'd chosen five novels from those twenty-five, and was going to learn how two young mothers—Casey and Angel—reacted to the representations of pregnant young women in them.

There were wreaths and red bows on the doors of Antic Granny's Antiques, the Country Home Gift Shop, and the Old Goat Bar, the well-kept brick-and-green-trim buildings that lined the touristy little downtown area of Alyssa; a plastic Santa perched on the old brick train depot in the center of the Alyssa Park Square, and a light snow dusted the ground.

I didn't know Casey and Angel well, but I hoped they would help me decide which novel we should read first. I asked Casey and Angel, both of whom were sitting in the back of the career room waiting for me, to look over the five books I had brought them. Turning *Like Sisters on the Homefront* (1995) in her hands, Angel said she liked the cover: "I don't know, I just like the way the girl looks." The cover of that novel shows a defiant-looking and very attractive young African American woman holding a big barefoot baby, who looks about two years old, against her hip. I was interested that Angel might be attracted to this image of a blue-jean-and-tee-shirted teenaged mother standing in a city scene. I wondered about the publishers and marketers of this text—who had they been imagining would read this wonderful novel, when they chose to draw the picture as they did? I didn't think they had someone like Angel—a white girl from rural schools in the middle of the country—in mind.

Casey was interested in *Mr. and Mrs. Bo Jo Jones* (1967), because I told her it was about a young couple who marry after they find out the girl is pregnant, and Casey was at that time settling into a new marriage as well as learning how to mother a baby. Both girls wrote down the names of these novels and said they planned to get them from the library.

Imani All Mine

At an early meeting, as we were still awkwardly trying to get to know each other, I read out loud part of Connie Porter's novel *Imani All Mine* (1999). I love this novel—the beauty and grace of its writing, the religiosity it suggests throughout. This is not a novel written expressly for young adults (although Porter has written novels for young people, most specifically the *Addy* books in the American Girl series); its implied reader is not necessarily a young person, though its heroine is fourteen; it is not a novel that focuses narrowly on a problem or is overtly didactic. In this 1999 ALA Best Young-Adult Novel of the Year winner, Porter presents a brave and thoughtful African American teen mother who carefully and conscientiously tries to raise her daughter well. With Tasha, the young mother who names her daughter Imani when her friend Eboni tells her the word means faith in "some African language" (7), Porter is clearly troubling the stereotype of the teen mother. At fourteen, Porter's character Tasha is a mother on welfare but she is also a girl who is on the honor roll, who has the strong moral sense that compels her not to abort this baby produced by a rape, and who is contemptuous of her mother's white boyfriend in part because he was once foolish enough to take drugs (100). Tasha mothers her daughter lovingly and shows confidence in her ability: "Even though I done had her just five months, I got things down right. It's what you call a routine" (1). She bravely continues school even though almost every day there she sees the boy who raped her.

Porter gives Tasha powers far beyond those society gives her, powers to use her imagination to sustain life: Tasha baptizes her daughter, turns that old ritual into one of her own: "I poured [water] gentle over the top of her head, and I say, Imani Dawson, I bless you in the name of the Father and the Son and Holy Ghost. I say it to her like I have the power to say it. Like I have the right to be the one that blessed her" (80).

I know that Elizabeth Ellsworth (1997) would remind me that "a teacher can open a book and begin to read aloud from it to students, but she can never know or control the sense that students will make of it" (67), but I also know that this novel was, to my mind, a better "teacher" than either of the two other books I read later with these girls (174), by which I mean not only that this novel's language was deep and graceful, not only that it spoke to a maturity in its readers, not only that it expressed ambiguity and complexity in the world it described, but also that I agree deeply with the complex and angry political stance the novel took.

This novel participates in the "society is wrong" discourse described by Kelly and Luttrell. *Imani All Mine* also participates in the "stigma is wrong" discourse: when, at the end of the book, Tasha decides to have a second child out of wedlock, this decision is presented as a hopeful one, not as the choice of a confused or bad girl, or a girl who is a product of a bad home, but as an expression of the triumph of youth over sorrow. This novel is the only one of all the twenty-five young-adult novels about teen mothers that I read that participates in this particular, teen-mother-affirming discourse. In this novel, Porter comments on the creative and loving and courageous ways her character and real women like her try to live good lives in neighborhoods filled with violence.

Perhaps some of my passion was evident as I read to Angel and Casey, there at the metallic table around which we settled our chairs. Perhaps Angel and Casey just felt relieved that they were not being asked to read themselves, but could sit and read along as they heard the words wash over them. I read out aloud this first time not only because I understand that students, even teenagers, need to be read to (Burke 2000; Trelease 2006) but also because instinctively, and from my own life, I know the pleasure of hearing texts read out aloud.

After I finished reading the first two chapters of the book to Casey and Angel, the girls talked about it with excitement and vibrancy in their voices. Casey said, "Fourteen. So, yeah, I was scared when I found out too, like she was too," and, later,

> It was smart of her not to get rid of the baby, not having an abortion. And then I thought it was smart of her to start going to those classes. I wish I would have done that. And I—just like Imani thought her baby had a routine before he was born I thought Russ did, too. Oh and she mentioned how her stomach didn't stick out all that much, mine did. It was way out to there.

Casey: And I know how she felt when her friend's mom would give her that look.

Cynthia: Ooh. You had people give you that look?

Casey: Ah yeah. It was hard. My parents, like 3 months before we got pregnant, they were always saying I don't want to be a grandparent. They knew way before me and Sam knew.

Cynthia: They could just tell.

Casey: Yeah. It was hard to hide it.

Angel: I wrote down some things . . .She was afraid to tell her mother, I was major afraid to tell mine. She didn't like how her body looked, I looked, oh God, I looked like a HORSE.

The girls were familiar with aspects of the story in *Imani All Mine*; having recently entered the world of teen motherhood, they were predisposed to be interested in and positive about this story. Eager to talk about their experiences—the bottles, late-night feedings, diapers, doctor visits, and the strange experiences of pregnancy and labor—they had background knowledge that may have made listening to and reading this novel easier than listening to and reading texts on other subjects; the girls seemed as if they could, to some extent, find themselves in Porter's description of Tasha (Vinz 2000).

I read a short section in which Tasha's mother takes her to a female doctor, who chastises her for being pregnant: "too many of our girls throwing they lives away, giving up on they futures," the doctor says (22). I wondered if Casey or Angel had experienced any prejudice from the doctors they saw when they were pregnant. Casey defended her doctor, saying he was a "Christian," but Angel said:

> Some people, yeah, especially, like—middling people, not real young people and not real old people but, like-middle-ish people—they look at me, like if I'm in the grocery store with Ben, like that doctor was to Tasha, like they think I'm a slut or something. Yeah.

The girls were excited about *Imani All Mine*; Angel copied down its name. Later she asked me its title again: "What book was that you read us last week?" And, when I told her I thought she could get it out of the library, she said, "You didn't make us copies?"

Make Lemonade

Some days after I read parts of *Imani All Mine* to them, I asked Casey and Angel to start reading *Make Lemonade* (1993) with me. I wanted the three of us to read together a book none of us had read before; I wondered how my being new to the novel would affect our conversation; I wondered if my ignorance of the novel would help us have conversations in which we created meaning together more than we had in our talk about *Imani All Mine*. Also, I had heard many positive comments made about *Make Lemonade*, its different structure—

it's written as a series of poems—its deracialized characters, its two lower-class protagonists. I thought it would be an easy read as well: My copy says it has been written for students in 5th through 12th grades.

Casey, Angel, and I had begun to get to know each other, and to be a bit of a group. I knew to expect them to be waiting for me in the back of the career center, or talking to Melinda, when I breezed in from my long cold drive up to Alyssa; they knew to expect me to take some time to pull myself together before we talked. The organizing of the tape recorder became a ritual that the girls helped me with; this was a way for them each to demonstrate competence and to show the importance of these dialogues to all of us.

During our conversations, Casey and Angel shared photos of their mothers, their homes, and their significant others; Casey suggested ways for Angel to get into programs, like Independent Living, that had been good for her. Shaking her head, Casey talked about friends of hers ("He was a good kid, but he was into drugs like meth, and that's why he died. I mean, nobody helped him, and that makes me so mad"); her past problems ("I was very suicidal for a long time, I mean, I overdosed, I took 30 pills of Prozac, all kinds of stuff") and her husband's family ("Sam's father is gay. Some people around here have problems with that, but I don't. And his boyfriend is Japanese"). She talked about her love of her son ("I'm so excited—I'm going to get Russ's footprint tattooed on my arm and Sam is going to get his hand and his footprint").

Angel talked about her boyfriend, Jason, and her wish that he would come back to her. She talked about other boys she was dating, too, though. She talked about Ben ("He's got a binky and a blanky. Gotta have 'em both"); and about her family back home in Alabama ("I lost my last grandma. Died of cancer. She cut her boob off but she died anyway. She never smoked or anything. She was so sweet").

Certainly Casey's life included a stronger support network than Angel's did—Casey had a husband who was generally helpful to her, a mother with whom she had a fairly understanding relationship now, at least one brother whom she considered to be an ally, and many troublesome and not-so-troublesome friends; Angel had a boyfriend she only sometimes saw, and who gave her trouble, and a mother who worked two part-time jobs and was not very attentive. Angel was by far the more vulnerable of these two young women.

In our conversations, the girls seemed to enjoy the fact that they had sometimes read farther than I had (**Angel:** Um, how far did you read? **Cynthia:** To chapter four. **Angel:** Should I explain what happens after that?). They seemed to feel comfortable when we all sat and read lines out aloud together, trying to figure out what was happening; and often, often, the conversation about the book veered off into other, more personal topics.

The Personal Reader

Angel: I get confused. I think that's good. And then I read on and I think about what I thought about what I was reading when I get confused.

Cynthia: How did you imagine what the people looked like? Or did you?

Angel: I didn't even think about it. Well I guess I thought the 14-year-old was very very skinny, not much meat on her, cause it says she was skinny. And I imagined this teen mom being an individual. Being one of a kind. 'Cause that's hard. And she's still trying.

Cynthia: What about the mother of the 14-year-old, Verna LaVaughn? Did you imagine her?

Angel: Yeah. Kind of mean, yet has a sensitive side. Because she—before she gets to know about this teen mom Jolly, that Verna LaVaughn is babysitting for, she's okay with it, she's very supportive, saying it's what you need to do. And then when it comes down to her actually finding out about the teen mom Jolly, she's very upset that Verna LaVaughn might be helping her too much but she kind of understands—kind of understands what kind of a situation Jolly's in but yet she doesn't want her daughter babysitting for her anymore. I think Verna LaVaughn's mom is just really supportive and she really didn't like it when Jolly lied to her.

In *Make Lemonade*, the main character, 14-year-old Verna LaVaughn, decides to babysit for Jolly, a teen mother, because she wants to earn money so she can go to college and get out of her building in which "in 64 apartments nobody ever went to college" (Wolf 1993, 10). Through working for Jolly, Verna learns a bit about what life is like for a teen mother, as she watches Jolly struggle with toilet training, with a job loss, with sexual harassment on the job, with a dirty house, and with bills. As working for Jolly becomes more and more difficult, and as Jolly becomes less able to pay Verna LaVaughn for her work, readers watch Verna live through a moral struggle, listening as Verna does some of what Andrew H. Miller (2002a) calls that "practical reasoning in which we accommodate and test fact and value, case and rule, in particular circumstances" (79). Throughout the novel Verna asks herself, and the reader, questions about how much she should sacrifice her goals to help someone who is less fortunate than she is. In this way, as we read this novel, we watch the "ethically burdened thought" (Miller 2002a, 79) of Verna and see how through that thinking she chooses who she will become. As Casey and Angel and I watched Verna make these decisions we, too, were making decisions: that attempt to create a "moral framework for living" that Ochs and Capps (2001) suggest occurs so often in narrative telling, that search for "right selfhood" that Bruner (2003, 77) says all our narratives conduct, occurs also as we read, or, as Miller (2002a) puts it: "watching others think could spur one to become oneself" (80).

The character Verna LaVaughn is a first-person narrator whose knowledge is limited; though she has power in that she is the teller and shaper of the story, unlike an omniscient narrator, she can only describe the limited knowledge that one person can have (Trites 2000, 71). Though Verna has a direct relationship with the implied adolescent readers of the novel (Trites 2000, 72), many of the values she relays are learned by both the reader and by Verna from Verna's mother, a character who sees some parts of the story that the main teller cannot. Verna's mother "voices the didactic ideology" (74) of the novel, through her conversations with and warnings to her daughter. Jolly initially rebels against the advice of Verna's mother, who seems to use her adult authority to repress and undercut the little power that Jolly has. Although I voiced some criticisms of Verna's mother, all of the young women liked and defended her. Angel in particular saw her as being "very caring." "She's going to help pay for the college a little bit," said Angel, "that's very very caring."

Verna's mother wields a power that undercuts the authority of her daughter's narrative voice, which perhaps also undercuts the power of the adolescent reader, implying as it does that only adults can have wisdom (Trites 2000, 79). Jolly brings herself out of powerlessness in part by following some of Verna's mother's suggestions. Jolly gains power also by aligning herself fully with the institution of school. In this novel succumbing to the power of the institution of school (Trites 2000, 33) is presented as the beginning of adult wisdom, and, unlike most schools outside of fiction, the school Jolly finally attends presents both girls with many kinds of help: not just a daycare center but a financial aid seminar (Wolf 1993, 118), a self-esteem class (86), an apprentice program (126), encouragement to go to college (118) as well as teachers (118) and counselors (124) who have plenty of time to help their students think through and solve their personal problems.

I asked Beth Manning to read this book; she said the book seemed outdated, especially in its depiction of the welfare system, to her. She didn't think teen mothers would accept the "quite stereotyped" image of the teen mother presented in the book. She found the book "sometimes aggravating, sometimes impressive, sometimes unrealistic."

The writer may be reflecting a very old view of accepting welfare, given her age. Reform came about in the 1960s, long before the setting of this book, I presume. I was on welfare in the 1970s and I did not have an aversion to the practical help that I so badly needed, nor did any of the moms I worked with in the 1980s and beyond.. My other issue is with the over-the-top caricature of the poor, illiterate, single mom that Jolly is. I have certainly known moms who had some of the problems that Jolly had but not all rolled together.

All of the young women who read this novel with me said that Jolly seemed to them to be true to life. Casey said:

> I know people just like that. This young guy Rich I knew, the boys' mom was in prison, I mean they had dishes stacked up to here and Rich didn't even give those boys a bath. I mean, it was just gross. There were times I'd come over and give them a bath. I mean, just like this girl in this book, it's really hard to be a young parent.

As I asked her to, Angel annotated her copy of *Make Lemonade*. On her copy she circled the words "drab" and "diagram," and wrote "don't know" beside them; after a line in the text that says "the tabs" of the teen mother's babysitting advertisement have not been taken by anyone, Angel wrote, "shows that a lot of people don't care about teen moms." After certain things the toddler character says, Angel wrote "cute!" At a different point Angel wrote "just like most friends—not supportive." In one paragraph the teen mother Jolly says "Reality is I got baby puke on my sweater and shoes/and they tell me they'll cut off the electricity/and my kids would have to take a bath in cold water/and the rent ain't paid like usual./reality is my babies only got one thing in the whole world and that's me and that's reality." Angel circled that paragraph and wrote "ain't that the truth."

None of the teen mothers who read this novel immediately identified with the teen mother Jolly, though, as they had identified with the teen mother who tells the story of *Imani All Mine*; primarily, when they read *Make Lemonade*, they identified with the younger, inexperienced girl, Verna, who is the first-person narrator of the story. The young women were, then, conventional readers, reading as the text asked them to. Because I was surprised that they didn't identify with the teen mother more than they did, I asked Angel directly about whether she saw herself as being like Jolly in any way. Angel answered,

> Oh, struggling, I guess, we're both struggling. Except I'm a lot neater. Except when it comes to my car and my bedroom. But—I don't have two kids, but I don't have a job, either. But like that girl I want to give Ben more than I can but I don't have a job so I know I can't.

The Helpless Reader

When he learned that Casey was reading *Make Lemonade* in a book club with me, her husband Sam asked her to read it out aloud to him every night. They liked this ritual, Casey said, because "It helps me calm down at the end of a long day." Her voice was relaxed and warm when she described this experience, and she seemed calmer, to me, when we had this conversation, than she had in the past. Maybe that was because Russell's ear infection had eased up and she was no longer up with him late nights, or maybe it was because she felt she was doing well at the project I had set before her. Maybe she sounded comfortable because she was talking, in this conversation, about her husband, of whom she was extremely proud.

Cynthia: Now I want you to tell me about reading *Make Lemonade* out aloud. Where were you sitting?

Casey: In my living room on my couch.

Cynthia: Were you sitting together on the couch?

Casey: Um-hm.

Cynthia: Um . . . what does it feel like to read to him?

Casey: Makes it easier because I—I—it's fun because if I don't understand something he's there to explain it to me and if I don't know a word either and it's, it's—I've never been able to read, I mean, especially out aloud.

Cynthia: You stumble over words, and you're slow?

Casey: And so, I mean, I feel really comfortable reading with him, it's a lot of fun, because I mean, he— he's very emotional (laughing) and so I mean he gets upset about—and then he'll get all excited—and then he'll get upset and y' know, it's just funny—

Cynthia: What did you—did you talk about the book at all?

Casey: He would ask me questions that he'd know the answer to already and he'd ask me just so I'd remember because I have a hard time remembering what I read.

Cynthia: But it's not like he corrects you it sounds like, it's not like reading with a teacher.

Casey: No, no.

Casey felt safe reading with her husband—it was different from her first reading experiences and different from school, in that way—and in the conversation above she laughed at her husband because he got 'so into it.' She didn't mind—all that much—when he asked her teacher-like questions about names and situations in the book to see whether she remembered them or not. In questioning Casey, of course, Sam used some of his college- and gender-earned power; and it is not surprising that his flexing of his intellectual muscles happens around the site of reading, which has so often been used as a tool for maintaining power.

They read sitting together on their couch, with their baby Russ in a car seat next to them. In describing her reading to me, Casey said she enjoyed how emotional her husband became at some parts of the book, for example

> when the baby gets the spider caught in her throat. I mean he was scared, he didn't want her to die . . . it was so funny, and he said why, it's not funny! But I kept reading, and he's like, why don't you go back, and I'm like, no! I want to find out! But he got all upset, he like, was almost crying. Russ was there next to us when I was reading and I could see Sam was thinking about him, about what could happen to him, just like when the baby almost died. I laughed at him but. . . I was getting kind of emotional too.

Casey and her husband were clearly feeling that "helplessness native to reading" that Andrew H. Miller (2002b) writes of when he describes readers who feel "perfectly helpless" as they watch characters make bad choices that will lead them or those they love to danger (81). Some part of Casey and Sam's intense reactivity to this scene in the novel—particularly Sam's tears—is an expression of that helplessness, and also of their growing awareness of their powerlessness as parents. As Casey and Sam read together they were aware of the many discourses that told them that young parents cannot possibly be good enough; they imagined what could happen to their baby son if they were not vigilant parents. Casey sometimes seemed irritated by the way in which the young-adult novels we read claimed to know who she was as a teen mother (Blackford 2004, 40). She made it clear that she did not see herself in Jolly and was not particularly interested in knowing her. But in this one case she seemed to experience no distance: She and Sam were right there with Jolly, experiencing the panic of having a baby who nearly chokes to death.

A Dance for Three

Some weeks after the group finished reading *Make Lemonade*, I read *A Dance for Three* (2000) by Louise Plummer with Angel, at her suggestion. When I called her from work to say happy birthday—she had just turned eighteen—Angel volunteered, "I read an interesting book myself, *A Dance for Three*. It's about a girl who gets pregnant. Her name is Hannah and the guy is Milo and she gets pregnant and waits three months to tell him and when she does he punches her right in the face. Then she goes crazy and is in a mental hospital. It's real good."

A Dance for Three is, as Angel suggested, a book about a girl in trouble. Written by a professor of English who says she decided to write the book when a relative of hers became pregnant out of wedlock, it strives to show how unwanted pregnancy can be related to a host of other problems a young person might be having. There is of course some truth to this idea that girls who get pregnant early are often girls with other problems: One of my teacher informants said that most of the five hundred teen mothers she had taught over the years had become pregnant after some tragedy had happened in their lives: "A grandmother died, there was a divorce, a serious breakup. It was amazing, the connections were so clear," this teacher said. This connection was confirmed in conversations with older teen mothers who, looking back, claimed that they started "acting wild" when their grandmother died or their father left home.

Seeking, I think, to show a teen mother in a compassionate and more complicated light, *A Dance for Three* speaks to this pattern of pregnancy after tragedy or loss, as none of the other books mentioned so far in this essay have. The character Hannah is dealing with grief over the death of her father, and with her mother's agoraphobic response to that death; she falls in love with the no-good, good-looking male character in the novel when he sings a song her father had sung to her (Plummer 2000, 35).

A Dance for Three is one of those books that participates primarily in the "wrong girl frame" (Kelly 2000, 47; Luttrell 2003, 27); like that discourse, the novel is complex because its author is trying to show compassion for the confused teenage narrator who makes some bad choices. This novel is also one that serves "both to reflect and perpetuate the cultural mandate that teenagers rebel against their parents" (Trites 2000, 69); it clearly presents Hannah's pregnancy as a form of deviance, and it shows the main character learning to accept the institutions—the family, the school, the mental hospital—that shape her life (69). This novel is clearly another "tool of socialization" (54) in which the narrator rebels by becoming pregnant and having a nervous breakdown and then, through the help of a surrogate mother figure (in this case a therapist), accepts the importance of institutions in her life, and becomes a person ready to accept conventional, adult life.

But the book is unusual in that it speaks to an issue none of the other young-adult novels I've read addresses: the pain an unwanted pregnancy can create for other members of the family. It is as if, in most of these books, the main characters' lives do not affect the lives of the people they live around. In *A Dance for Three*, however, the brother of the father of the baby goes to see it in the hospital and mourns its loss when it's adopted, saying that "Uncles have no rights" (Plummer 2000, 218). One of the older women I spoke to for my study, Jennifer, who became pregnant out of wedlock when she was in high school, told me that her brother's reaction to her baby was a major force in her decision to keep her child:

> There was no way I had any idea what a parent was, I had no idea. And so honest to god I had the papers signed and everything. I thought, when I went to the hospital, that I was giving him up. For adoption. They wouldn't let me see him because of that. But my brother came, he's younger than me, and he had seen him, and he said, well you're going to keep him, aren't you? And I just said, yeah I think I am, and he goes, oh, good, and he really felt so glad, and I think he thought it would be more like a brother for him. And then I got to see him, and that's how I made that decision.

Few of the young-adult novels I've read about teen parents capture the appreciation and regret some of the young mothers I've spoken with express about their decision to keep their children.

Angel seemed to like *A Dance for Three* in part because it retained a violent quality that seemed true to her life. I think she also liked the book because it helped her present her identity to me, an identity that was very much wrapped up in being a teen mom. She liked talking to me about this book because it helped promote that sense of knowledge and authority that becoming a teen mother had given her.

When I asked her which, of all of the pregnant teens she had read about in our time together, she "identified" with most, she talked about the reality she found in *A Dance for Three*:

> In this one—Hannah? Because like in that one I thought everything was going to be perfect with Jason and stuff and then we fought all the time and the first time I told him he was like, are you sure if it was his, just like Milo in that book. He lied about me and said no I never had sex with her. And Milo beat her up. I related to that part, too, because Jason and me have been in quite a bit of fights. Never to the point where I had to go to the hospital but almost! I pressed charges against him but then I dropped them but he had to stay in jail for one day.

When I asked Angel why she had dropped the charges against her boyfriend Jason, she said, "Well, I love him. He doesn't want to be with me. Well, he acts

like he wants to be with me but he doesn't act like he wants to be with me?"
The character Hannah in *A Dance for Three* expresses bewilderment similar—
though nowhere near as moving—to the bewilderment Angel expresses here.

The character Hannah has many more supports than Angel had, and her
violent boyfriend—though he doesn't come to much grief in the novel—is
scolded for his bad behavior by the author in ways Angel's boyfriend most
likely will never be. One of the pleasures of reading fiction, I suppose, is that
we can see people get what they deserve.

Considerations about the Reading

Though Casey and Angel were able to critique the stereotypes of teen
mothers that they were aware of out in the world—as evidenced by Angel's
comments on how other people reacted to her and her son in the grocery store—
neither of them commented on stereotypical aspects of the representations of
teen mothers in these novels. A teacher would need to help Casey and Angel
begin to critically consider the ideology of these texts, and to see how they
were being positioned as readers, by, in particular, the novel *Make Lemonade*,
to critique the teen mother figure. A teacher would need to help the young
women try to locate discourses of female teenage sexuality in these novels as
well (Coffel 2002, 16). Though many young adult novels about teen mothers
do not describe the financial difficulties some teen mothers experience, or the
particular problems of single parenting, they do, according at least to Angel and
Casey, capture some aspects of two teen mothers' real lives. Among these are
the pleasure and strangeness of a changing body, the sense of condemnation
from others, the joys and troubles of new responsibility, and the violence of
some teen relationships.

Though Casey and Angel later read parts of *Detour for Emmy* and *Annie's
Baby* with me, their responses to these novels were, like the responses described
above, quite personal and uncritical; they recognized the cruel boyfriend
figures right off, they saw what was coming toward the end of *Annie's Baby*, and
they identified with the first-person narrator of these novels rather uncritically.
They enjoyed the novels, and the novels did seem to provide a sense of
community-through-reading for them, some sense that they were not alone in
their experience of being teen mothers (Coffel 2002). Still, they weren't able—
at least in our short meetings—to pick out the pernicious ideology in some of
these novels, even when I tried to draw their attention to it.

I wonder as I write these words about the "violence" of the representations
of the teen mothers in these texts (Ellsworth 1997, 126). What readings of

young mothers' stories have been foreclosed by these texts? In reading these young adult novels, Angel and Casey were in many ways provided with stories they had heard before, stories they were living in and against and through. I wonder what this reading has let loose in the world (126), what new in these young women's minds has happened because of our readings of these conservative and new, unimaginative and rich, deeply meant and overly simple young-adult novels.

Chapter 5

The Happy Rainy Day: Teen Mothers and Teachers Writing

Like the teachers Wendy Atwell-Vasey interviews for her book *Nourishing Words*, (1998) I have always been the kind of person who "writes about love" (Atwell-Vasey 1998, 21) when I write about reading and writing. For me, writing has always been a "vehicle to a deeper, more nuanced sense of [myself] as a being in the world" (Yagelski 2009, 15); unlike Casey, Angel, Brenda, and Gabriel, I have always used writing as a way of caring for myself. How can my sense of literacy, so closely woven into my sense of self, be of use to young women who have primarily experienced a school-bound literacy, which sees a student-written text through a focus on correctness? Robert Yagelski (2009, 16) suggests that we might begin by teaching teachers and students to value the writer's *experience* when writing, even more than her writing process or the correctness of her finished product.

Beth Manning described a conversation with a teacher at the Thomas Jefferson Learning Center who seemed to value appropriateness of language over an earnest expression of thought and feeling.

> One of my long-term part-time instructors came in to grump about a student's essay that she thought showed laziness. She didn't like the fact that he used what she called swear words. I said it looks to me like what he's writing amongst the swear words are some really impassioned opinions about the war, about where this country's going, about how he feels alienated by this country. I think that you're reading somebody's honest heartfelt thoughts. I think you can ask him to tone this stuff down, but I think this is just the way he sees it.
>
> And then I talked to him about it. I explained it as a problem of his being heard. I said I believe that your teacher can't see what you're saying through all the obscenities. And he was really embarrassed. She was upset that he had said something rude about the president. And he was so embarrassed that she had not understood what he was saying through his words.

Similarly, perhaps, to the young man Beth described, Brenda explained with her usual exuberance the ways her composition classes at Thomas Jefferson are teaching her standard English, which she believed will allow her to be heard more readily by others:

And see in composition they had to teach us how to say proper words like, *is, was*, past tense, present tense. That was interesting because that's a lot of stuff that you need to carry on. You're not gonna write "my dad and me are going to the . . ." I mean you hear people say that and you wanta correct them. I mean *I* want to correct them but you don't want to be rude and stuff. Because I remember I used to not say nothing like that! But I remember how I used to say something—I can't remember what word I used to say—no—I know—*swum* instead of *swam*, I used to say that, and I always used to get corrected on that and I remember getting frustrated when everybody corrected me on certain things like that. So when people say those things I don't correct them. I just think if they want to go back to school they can learn that.

The ways these two above use writing is for a more public purpose than the one I suggested Casey and Angel use. I wanted to try to focus on the value of their experience of writing more than "the obsession with form and correctness that characterizes school-sponsored writing." I wanted, in asking them to write for me, to allow Casey and Angel to begin to understand "writing as an inquiry into self and world" (Yagelski 2009, 16).

During the times Casey, Angel, and I met to read and talk about young-adult novels, I asked them to write for me. Both had annotated chapters of the novels we read, and both had written to the prompt, "Other people think I am . . . but I know I am . . . " suggested by my readings of Wendy Luttrell's book, *Pregnant Bodies, Fertile Minds* (2003). Casey's answer to this prompt had been a long paragraph. She said she'd asked her husband and mother to tell her what they thought about who she was, and that she'd typed the paragraph on her home computer late at night. Her paragraph was shaped almost like a poem:

> My friends and family all say about the same thing about me. They say that I am very smart but very bad at spelling. I have my good moments and bad. My mother and husband say that I am way to hard on myself. I often say that "I can't do this!", "I'm not a good mom!" and "I never have time for anything!" Along with that, they say that my expectations are very high. If its not done, my way its not right. I try way to hard to get everything perfect. Frustrated is a big thing with me, my husband said. My mom says that I get frustrated at the smallest things. Part of the reason I get so flustered is that I worry about everyone else's problems. However, all and all they say that I am happy person most of the time.

Thinking about Casey's life as she described it to me, I was interested that she expressed her identity as being deeply embedded in the lives of her family; I was impressed as well, given the life history she told me, that she can see herself—or say that her family sees her—as a happy person most of the time.

In her answer to the same question, Angel wrote a simpler response:

My friends: think I want to get back together with Jason—they're wrong! Other people like adults think I'm not a good mother to Ben—they're wrong! I think: I'm a good mother to Ben!

I asked both girls to write their life stories as a way, in part to get to know them, and as a way to see their writing. Casey brought her autobiography to me but Angel never did. Casey's written story is different from the stories she told me in conversation:

I was born in 1983. My parents' names are John and Susan Walter. I have an older brother Joe. He is six years older than me

When I was five my parents got a divorce. They had a two-year custody battle. I ended up in foster care for about two years because of the abuse from my father. I got to go back and live with my mom.

Shortly after I got back home, my mom married Bill Barnes. They had two kids, Deborah and Mikey. My life was hard with Bill as my new father because he would abuse me at night while mom was sleeping. There was nothing I could do about it. In 90 they were divorced.

In 95 my mom met this man, who I dearly hated at the time. I got another sister in March of that year. Then in March of 97 my mom and Alex got married.

I was not a very good teen. I made life for my parents a living hell. Finally, I ended up in Shott County Youth Shelter for a few months. Then I ended up going back a few months later. Since I was almost 18 my worker and I talked about doing a program called Independent Living. I got to do the program and got my own apartment in Alyssa.

I started to date Tom; he was 21 years old. The relationship was very bad. There were lots of drugs and parties. In addition, along with all that there was more abuse. I stayed with Tom for two years because I was afraid of what may happen to me if I left.

I started working at Stanleys and I fell in love with my manager Sam. I loved working there. The work was fun. I loved the customers, they always made me smile. The only time I felt safe was when I was at work and Sam was there.

In November of 2000, we found out that my mom had breast cancer. At this time, my mom and I were not getting along. But that changed fast. She needed me and I needed her. I was so scared that I was going to lose her. Sam was the only one I could talk to about it. She went through chemotherapy and radiation. After 9 long months, she had her hair back and was cancer free.

October 2, 2002 Sam and I were married in a beautiful ceremony with all our friends and family there. We have just moved into a cute two bedroom apartment not far from my mother. I helped my mom with her daycare and with my brothers and sisters. Sam got a job at Menards where he continues to work today. I still help out my mom.

November 14, I had a beautiful baby boy. He was the best thing that ever happened to me. He is a very good baby. He sleeps through the night and seldom cries. I've thought about having more children some day, but after visiting Mom and my siblings and listening to them argue, I've been rethinking it.

Married life and motherhood have not been easy for me. It is a big adjustment. I was just learning how to take care of myself and now I have much more responsibility. It's often difficult dealing with a spouse and his needs. We do argue, but we always make up. Many disagreements are about money and chores. I don't know how my mom did it!

Reading this autobiography of Casey, I wonder what she has left out because it didn't seem appropriate to a woman's story; I wonder what pieces of that conventional female fiction of becoming she's appropriated here. I notice that, differently from the stories she told me in conversation, this written story begins and ends with her mom, with her mother's marriages, her mother's illness, and her new appreciation for the difficulty of her mother's life. I remember how Casey said, about the women who took care of her during the years when, because of her father's abuse, she didn't live with her mother, "When I'm out shopping, or walking around with Russell, I'm always running into my foster moms; I see them around town all the time." She said, "It was hard for my mom to be away from me, I know; I know she used to cry every night."

Many people have commented on the value of the personal writing I was asking Casey and Angel to do, the sort of writing I have done most of my life, in diaries: writing as a kind of caring for the self. This internal making-sense-of-the-world type of writing is mentioned by Judith Musick (1993) in *Young, Poor, and Pregnant* as "the metacognitive practice of putting words to things" (230), which can help a teen mother "master" an emotional experience, and use language to "put a psychological space between feeling and action. It encourages reflection and self-awareness, thinking before automatically doing" (230). Carol Johnson, one of the teachers I interviewed for this book, a woman who had taught teen mothers in the Midwest for over fourteen years, had also discovered that writing can be used as a way to capture and explore the self:

I want them to use their journals as a therapeutic venue. They don't always have someone who will listen to them, so if they can put their thoughts down on paper and then sometimes, later, they reflect on them and they'll see, gee I was so mad about such and such a thing last Thursday and here it is this Thursday and that's not even an issue any more . . .

It's a truism that writers write best about subjects they are most interested in; if conversation was any indicator, Casey and Angel were still fascinated by the experience of giving birth, by the strange "inside story" of pregnancy, that experience of "two people living under one skin" (Luttrell 2003, 4), that new relationship of the self to the body that the experiences of pregnancy and childbirth created. I expected that they would write well about the experience of birth. I thought as well that, as with telling the narrative of their lives verbally, writing this story out might provide Angel and Casey with the opportunity to reshape or reframe the experience, giving them some perspective on it, and helping them make some internal sense of what must have been one of the most powerful experiences of their lives.

The Happy Rainy Day in November by Casey

> It was very early in the morning at about 5:30, when I got up to go to the bathroom like normal. As I was getting back into bed I noticed my leg was wet. Sam called the Doctor. We got everything together and we were on our way.

> When we arrived at the hospital it was like going to a hotel. The room had a big TV and everything that came with it. Sam got to eat breakfast. I thought it would be hard to see him eat but it was very easy. I was way too happy to eat knowing that my baby is almost here.

> I wasn't able to walk like most women can. The baby's head wasn't down far enough. I had to stay in bed all day. I had lots of visitors all day, my parents and my sisters and my sister in law.

> It was a rainy afternoon but nothing but sunshine inside. My whole family thought that I would be very irate. But to their surprised I was very happy and pleasant. The Doctor gave me some pain meds and I fell right to sleep. I slept for a few hours and when I woke I got my epiderale. It was rainy out but I was still very happy. I knew with every contraction, it was a minute closer to seeing my baby.

> The evening was finally here and it was time to push, so I said! My parents had left to go get something to eat. I needed them, and Sam wanted to what just a little bit. That was the only time I got a little mad. So Sam called them and they were on their way. When my parents arrived I had been pushing for about 30 minutes.

> The baby's head was almost out and the Doctor let me feel the head. That was the greatest moment in my life. An hour later I got my baby boy! All I did was scream that: I GOT MY BABY BOY, I GOT MY BABY BOY! Over and over again. When I finally got to hold him, he felt like he weighed a million pounds. It was the happiest rainy day ever!

> RUSSELL XXX XXXXX Weigh 9# Length 21 inches

When I asked Casey to tell me what writing this had felt like to her, she said she was amazed that the story had turned out so short. "I thought I'd just write pages and pages, I was worried that it would come out too long," she said. "I could write lots more about this but—I don't know. What I like about it is that it was a rainy day and I like how I say that. It was real rainy, but me and Sam were really happy."

Yagelski (2000) troubles the idea of the lone "Romantic Writer," suggesting that the process of writing may not be such a lonely one after all. Yagelski relates the common "Romantic ideal of the inspired writer" to "American cultural beliefs in individualism and self-determination" (72). Yagelski suggests that not only is the idea of the lone writer incorrect, but that, because of thinkers like Michel Foucault and Claude Lévi-Strauss, the notion of the single individual has been troubled (Yagleski 2000, 73). Just as postmodernism has questioned the reality of the single, coherent individual, any written work created is also created out of multiple strains, the "product of existing discourses within which the book's meanings are determined" (73).

Yagelski (2000) suggests that teachers might be helped by seeing their students as people who are negotiating and struggling with various, sometimes contradictory, discourses as they write. This stance might help teachers see that what they would have called errors might be difficulties related to students' efforts to negotiate among competing discourses (84).

What were some of the discourses about teenaged mothering that Casey struggled within and against as she wrote "A Happy Rainy Day"? Clearly the text itself is an argument, an insistence that on the rainy day of her son's birth "everything was sunshine inside." This is of course the way a woman is expected to feel on the arrival of her child—and it's surely how Casey felt about the birth of her son. And yet this conventional response is also contrary to the response others might expect of a 19-year-old who has just recently married the father of her child: the mother might be chagrined, embarrassed, alone, and lost, as some of the young women in the young-adult stories I read with Casey are when they have their children. So this story plays with and complicates the discourses that make it up (Yagelski 2000, 78). Casey is showing some of the agency she has within the discourses that make up her writing.

Influencing Casey's story as well are the many-years-old stories that women tell of birthing: "I wasn't able to walk like most women are," writes Casey, and one can imagine all the stories she has heard and read about the birthing experiences of her sisters, her mother, her sister-in-law who huddle around her bed in this essay. This essay might have been influenced as well by those discourses still alive in the United States that suggest that the birth of a boy is an event more special than the birth of a girl ("I got my baby boy! I got my baby boy!"). There is also a certain sense, finally, in which this essay participates in the discourse of fairy tales—the hospital room is "like a hotel" with a big TV and "everything that went with it," her parents come to see the baby's birth, and, one can almost sense that fairy godmothers might be there, too. The title of the essay is a little like a fairy tale as well, or like a children's story. (I think of *The Happy Egg* or *Happy Marbles!* from Ruth Krauss's classic collection *Somebody Else's Nut Tree.*)

In this short essay, Casey is trying to "write herself into that American fable of success" (179) by showing that "everything was sunshine inside." In order to write herself into that fable, according to Yagelski (2000), Casey must also "accept the terms by which she is defined within the discourses of American education and of American capitalist culture, terms that can be seen as limiting her in the first place" (179). Casey cannot write about herself as a member of a certain group of young women who have been introduced to sex early, and therefore marry early; she cannot write about herself as one of many people whose choices have been constrained by gender and lack of access to middle-class power; rather, in order to write herself into that fable of American success she must present herself as an individual, entirely free of the influences of power, class, psychology, or gender.

There is very little vulnerability in this writing: Casey is saying, as she does so insistently in person: nothing's the matter here. Perhaps Casey writes the way she does about the birth of her baby because she realizes she has another hold on her man, and thus anticipates a more stable future than she's had in her past; perhaps she writes so happily because she feels that her identity will no longer be fragmented, but that she will be comfortably purposeful with the role, with the new identity, of mother; perhaps she writes so happily simply because she has that need for a "tidy" (Ochs & Capps 2001, 223) resolution to the complicated life story she told me. Perhaps she writes so happily simply because she is happy.

My reading of Casey's essay has also been influenced by my own experiences and by the discourses about mothering and teen mothering that surround me. I read Casey's essay as a mother who considers the birth of her son as one of the high points of her life; I read Casey's essay as a writer with a liking for narratives that, as Thomas Newkirk (1997), puts it, take a "turn" (12) and that suggest the "malleability of the self" (21); that have a clear "disjunctive illuminating moment, before-and-after an experience" (22) as Casey's essay does—before my baby boy came, after my baby boy came; I read Casey's essay as one enough familiar with the discourses of the academy to appreciate the aesthetic style that Newkirk calls "emotional displacement" (35), the lack of sentimentality, the understated quality, and the edge of humor ("I got very irate") that this short narrative provides. I read this text as one influenced enough by the discourses surrounding teen motherhood to notice Casey's capitalization of the word "doctor" (which feeds into the discourse that says that, though doctors are important people to all pregnant women, to younger, poorer, and more vulnerable teen mothers, doctors must seem like powerful authority figures); to notice Casey's statement that her room was like a hotel (which feeds into the discourse that says that teen mothers probably have less experience of the world than other people, and that having a baby may make them feel special); and to remind myself that when Casey writes "parents" she really means her fifth stepfather and her mother.

Finally, I appreciate the wonderful, portentous complexity of Casey's statement at the end of her narrative—a complexity that, to me, signals Casey's maturity and intelligence, her sense that her story may not be as happy as she suggests—her statement that "when I got to hold him, he felt like he weighed a million pounds." Casey's story describes, perhaps, the happy but not uncomplicated taking on of a huge responsibility. Casey may also be describing a joy much less complicated than I'm making it—a nine-pound baby would feel pretty heavy in a mother's arms, especially after a long labor.

Angel's narrative about the birth of her son—an untitled piece, with Angel's spelling mistakes replicated here—is quite different from Casey's:

> I knew I was pregnant because I missed my period. I went and bought a pregnancy test and it came out positive. I called Jason on the phone right after I found out and the right thing he said was "Are you sure" I told him yes and told him about the test. He told me he wanted me to take another test. The next day we got together and bought another test and went to Taco Bell. We ordered are food and then I went to the bathroom and took it. It came out positive. I put it in my purse and showed it to him. We talked about how to tell are parent! I wanted to tell them with both of us there but he didn't. He thought that it would be better for us to do it separated so we did. We went to the mall and I bought my mom and her boyfriend Barry gifts. When I got home mom was on the computer and Barry was at work. I pulled up a chair by my mother and told her I was pregnant. She said "You better not be." I said "I am!" I went upstairs for the rest of the night.
>
> The next day we talked about it and she asked me if I was sure. I told her "I have taken two pregnancy test and both were positive." I showed her the test! She looked at them for awhile then said "I want you to take one at a doctors office." I told her "I'll go to Birth Right" That was all that was said! Jason and I got together the next day and went

to Birth Right. Jason waited in the car while I went in. I had to fill out a sheet of paper about myself! While I was waiting to find out the Answer to if the test was positive or not I told the lady that I have take two home test and that they were both positive! I told her how my mother wanted me to come here and take one. She told me it was positive. She gave me a book "What to expect when your expecting," a pair of booties and a little plastic baby at like 6 weeks. I said thank you and she said a preyer with me and give me her number and told me to call her if I ever needed anything! I said thank you again and went back to the car! Jason knew what the test said as soon as I got into the car with all the stuff I had!

I didn't start showing til about 6 months. I never got sick or anything! I was getting huge and fast. By the time I was 9 months pregnant I had gained 50 pounds. I went to the doctors when I was told to. Never miss any! Everything was fine! The baby inside of me got the hiccup a lot and kicked me in the ribs a million time a day! Jason was great always rubbing, kissing, and talking to the unborn baby.

I got to the point that I was five days overdue! Mom had been making me go to work with her to make sure nothing happened to me! She always told me that walking would move thing along, so I went to the gym and walked on a treadmill for an hour! I drove back to my mothers work place and not even twenty minutes later I started to have contractions! I timed them for an hour and then called the doctor! They told me to time them for one more hour and if they are five minutes apart to come in to the hospital. She said if there not to call back to say what to do! I timed them for thirty minutes and they where like 4 to 5 minutes apart! Mom got to leave earlie to take me to the hospital!! I took us forty five minutes to get to the hospital! When we got there they took me to a room and gave me a gown! After I got into the gown they checked my servicks and told me I was one centimeter dilated and told me to walk up and down the hall for two hours so I did. When they checked me again I was still one centimeter dialated. They told me to go ahead and go home! Mom asked the nurse how long she thought it would be before I would need to come back! She told my mom it would more than likely be anywhere from 2 to 48 hours. Mom and I left to go home and Jason left to go to him brothers. Mom and I got about 5 to 10 minutes away and my water broke! Mom asked me if I was sure it was my water and that I didn't just pee. I told her I was sure! Mom turned around and I called Jason and told him to turn around because my water broke. I also called Barry and told him to bring Nicole "my little sister" to the hospital! When we got back to the hospital I told them what had happened. They checked me again. I was 2 centimeters!

My pains were getting worse and coming closer together! A few hours went by and I was 4 centimeters a couple more hourse went by I was 6 centimeters. My contractions were getting worse so I got a shot of newboare! I rocked in a rocking chair through my pains! Not long after that (a few more hours) it was time! My baby didn't want to come out. He came out a little and then right back in! Finally he came out! He was so beautiful! I had a pretty easy delivery!

It was 7:15 when he was born. He was 7 lbs 2 oz and 21 inches ½ inches long! The

nurses took him away for awhile to run test and everything so I got some sleep! When
I got up I held him for a long time!

The End!!

Angel's story is much more detailed, or (as she might say) "detailish," and
told with less awareness of a reader's needs than is Casey's; it is less carefully
shaped, and the details included are picked with less purpose. Similarly, Angel
shows less agency in working against the discourses about teen mothers that
surround her than Casey does: where Casey seems to be arguing against some
of our received ideas about what it's like for a teen to give birth, Angel's essay
is more conventional; some aspects of her story parallel the young-adult novels
that we read together.

As I read Angel's story, I see a confluence of the private and the public, the
commercial and the intimate. The private experience of discovering that she
is pregnant happens, for Angel, in the public and commercial space of Taco
Bell; Angel and Jason react to the discovery of her pregnancy by immediately
taking off to the mall to buy presents that will, they hope, offset the bad news
they will tell their parents. The brutal consumer economy enters the story in
other ways as well: in Angel's story the fact that her mother, a bartender at the
local country club, gets to take time off work to help her daughter give birth
deserves two exclamation points.

In Angel's story, I hear for the first time some of the language of the pro-
life movement, as when Angel writes about the "unborn baby," and when
the woman at Birth Right prays with Angel, who leaves the building with her
arms full of "stuff" the woman at Birth Right has given her. I also hear the
familiar story of the reluctant boyfriend—a story that is played out often in
the young-adult novels we read together—who doesn't want to believe that his
girlfriend is pregnant, and is too cowardly to take responsibility for his part in
the pregnancy, refusing to go with his girlfriend even to talk to her parents.

Finally, I wonder about all of the exclamation points that Angel uses in her
essay. As I read Angel's essay, because I share the academic sense of aesthetics
that appreciates understatement, Angel's use of exclamation points suggests
to me that her perspective on her son's birth is not one of "moral seriousness"
(Newkirk 1997, 96). At the same time I know, because I know the girl, that
Angel did take the birth of her son seriously. About her son Angel said:

Was having him a mistake? No. I'd rather have Ben than have half the stuck up people
that I used to be friends with. I would rather be Ben's mother and Ben's friend than
to go out with people who just—don't give a hoot. . . I know it's kinda—weird—me

being only 16 at the time. I guess- I wanted Ben because I wanted someone to care for cause my life was pretty much nothing, y' know, all I did was party and everything and I wanted to actually get away from everything. And I wanted to actually be able to take care of somebody because I love babies and one of these days I'm not going be living, something could happen today, something could happen tomorrow, something could happen in ten years and you know I wanted to—not take that chance. I didn't tell my mom I didn't want him, but I told her—he was a mistake. But that's not true, he wasn't a mistake. I say he was a miracle. I say he was a gift.

Conclusions

The last time Casey and Angel and I met for the Teen Moms' Book Club, it was the end of May. Geraniums and pansies swung in baskets outside of Antic Granny's Antiques and the Country Home Gift Shop; the ground around the Old Goat Bar and the mattress factory was muddy. On the long drive up from my hometown, grass was more yellow than brown; I saw swallows against the blue sky.

The girls were both beginning to lose some interest in meeting with me, I think. After our last meeting, Angel called finally to say that she couldn't come anymore because she had landed a waitressing job; Casey told me, the last time the Teen Moms' Book Club met, that the gym she and her mother had been trying to find funding for was ready to open, and that it would need to be her focus for a while.

The tiny reading-and-writing group I ran suffered the problems that plague many out-of-school book groups—the girls came late or not at all, some times they had not read the book, or had only read part of the book. Often, Casey and Angel were more interested in talking to me about what Barton and Hamilton call "ruling passions" (as cited in Luttrell & Parker 2001, 235–347)—in the case of these young women, this meant their children and their boyfriends—than they were in talking about reading, or the texts that I had asked them to read.

In *Landscape for a Good Woman* (1986) Carolyn Steedman refers to the fortitude and grit she developed when, as a working-class girl, she was told she would have to earn her own way through life. Steedman suggests that, finding that no one was telling stories about a working-class girl like herself, the fortitude that had been trained into her helped her to "go out and write [my story] for myself." Casey and Angel did not find themselves, exactly, in the stories that we read, stories that were not written for poor girls, or for girls who were mothers already. Casey and Angel were very conscious of the difference between the people they thought they were and the people others saw them as—the unwed pregnant teen on the teen parent panel, the overwhelmed young mother in the grocery store. Although Yagelski shows us how no one is ever, really, able to write a story that is entirely their own, and though Casey and Angel were only beginning to shape their stories, in their writing at least, they were consciously pushing against those old and too-often-told narratives about teenage motherhood; they were beginning, I think, to see how they might one day move, with grit and fortitude, toward writing stories they could call their own.

Utah, 1980:
Famous Mothers and Others

January 15

Liz Rosenstein suggested I break my classes into three- or nine-week chunks; that's helped me organize, and in my regular English class I'm taking Dainty's advice, and teaching writing other than "Young Goodman Brown." On the weekend I made mimeographed copies—23—of a play called *A Taste of Honey*, about an unmarried working-class girl who gets pregnant; for the next three weeks we'll read it aloud and write about the girl's mother in that play, and what qualities they think a good mother should nurture in herself.

Liz says I have to learn to *sell* what I'm teaching, and that I have to find energy to do things with the girls, take them out of the school, let the community be the teacher. And another thing, she said, no matter what you do, you're always teaching them something. What do you want to teach them? They like best the teachers who teach them what they feel they need to know.

But it really is getting better: Toya wanted to do her love poetry homework even though she'll get no credit; Carrie Johnson told me she's learning more in my dreams class than in any of her other classes. In Health yesterday, my student Ebony looked real sad and stayed after class and talked about how inadequate she feels, as a mother, as a student. She never has time both to do her schoolwork and care for her two kids well. There's dirty laundry all over her house, she said, in tears. Her boyfriend wants her to move to Nigeria with him, but she doesn't want her daughters to be away from their grandmother. I gave her my copy of *How to Be Your Own Best Friend*, and when I came into class this morning, there was a piece of strawberry cake sitting on my desk.

January 20

When the minister's wife who teaches down the hall told me she was pregnant, instead of congratulating her, I asked, "On purpose?"

January 22

Walking past the drugstore I chatted with some boys from Utah High School. When I told them I taught at the Teen Moms' Program they said, "Oh, that's not a real school." What do they think a "real" school is?

A continual issue for me here is just how lenient to be. Liz says the main thing we have to teach alternative-school-type kids is responsibility. Alice Haynes asked if she could take a spelling test over and I said no but I know she's just found out she's pregnant again and that would cause her to be thinking about other things.

I am basically doing all that I can to get them through. But then I do believe many students in my English class will flunk. And I don't believe I am by any means being too difficult. Boring, maybe. Requiring a lot of writing, certainly. But not requiring difficult work of them, perhaps not difficult enough. Then again, as Liz says, does the work have to be difficult for students to be learning?

January 27

Started an English elective on comparative religions two weeks ago. Some of the girls have been excommunicated from the Mormon church; they must be interested in this stuff. Maybe I should have read them excerpts from that book, *Isn't One Wife Enough?*

Took them to the Buddhist temple today: three gold altars covered with apples, oranges, and roses and the Rev. Suekawa explaining that Buddhists don't believe in God, exactly. Afterward Carrie, hanging around my room, telling me her mother wants to be a race car driver and is "real messed up," and saying, "You've kind of had a hard time this year, haven't you, Cindy?" This from a fifteen-year-old mom who has never missed a day of school, who works 30 hours a week doing bookkeeping so she can support her daughter Tiffany and the two of them can "be a family."

February 1

Brandy had a 7-pound girl yesterday, Josepha Lynn.

A woman came in to talk about home birth. She showed two films of women having their babies at home with family around, and how the father and the baby bond. Pregnant Rachel raised her hand and asked if fathers who attend the births of their children beat them less often.

February 11

Yesterday Tyra turned to my English class, gestured at me, and said, "Hey, you guys, she's been in school for *twelve years* and she STILL like writing!"

But I am exhausted. Some days I come home at 3 and sleep until morning. I have a little group of students who like my English electives, now: they've taken my three-week dreams course, my love poetry course, and my vocabulary course. They asked if my next English elective could be about teenage troubles. Teenage troubles! Don't we have enough of those around here? But I'm doing it—I had a social worker come in last week to list the warning signs of depression; I'm looking for someone to talk about dating violence. Tomorrow I'm planning to read the girls this case study of Sarah, which is partly based on memories of myself at their age:

> *Sarah is tired of hearing her mother and father fight. She broke up with her boyfriend and she's stopped going to school; she doesn't want to see her friends anymore. She never washes her hair or cleans her clothes because she's tired. Who is there to care? Lately she's been taking her parents' bottle of gin to bed with her —she drinks and takes a few pills to help her go to sleep each night.*
>
> *What can Sarah do to help herself?*
>
> *Where can she go for help or counseling? (Put a list of counseling services on the board as the girls suggest them.)*

February 12

After I read the piece about Sarah out loud in class, I said, "Write letters to Sarah, guys, tell her what to do, give her some advice." Maybe they'll see how they can use reading and writing as therapy, I thought; maybe helping out a girl in a situation like theirs will help them help themselves sometime. But the girls started talking and spilled out their stories to me: Susan King, who wants to be a psychologist, told me she tried to kill herself, shoving her hands through the glass of the hospital window after her daughter was born. Susan described how it felt to get her fingers sewn up after that, and how they don't really work right anymore. "Before I was married my hands were okay," she said. "Let's see . . . that was in ninth grade . . ."

Rosie Jaramillo is the girl the history teacher wishes could go to law school, she was so tough and quick as prosecutor in the mock trial against Utah High. She's eighteen, five-months pregnant, the mother of a two-year-old already. She's so smart that I find her quickness and insight unsettling. "I was just like that Sarah, Cindy," she said. "I wanted to kill myself. I got pregnant with Carrie on purpose, I know I did, I was real messed up. I needed a reason to live."

Rosie handed in a long letter, the first of her writing I've seen, and two weeks later, when we were on to other things, tough Rosie came up to me and asked, "Cindy? Whatever happened to that girl Sarah? Is she okay? I wrote a real good letter to her, I spent a lot of time on it. Did it help? Is she okay? Did she get counseling?"

How to explain that I had made Sarah up? But I am beginning to love some of these girls.

Chapter 6

Schoolgirls:
Before, During, and After Pregnancy

In some ways the Teen Moms' Program was a school that Nel Noddings (1992, 14) would say provided "caring and continuity for students." Unlike the Alyssa and Thomas Jefferson Learning Centers, and unlike most schools, it was a place that foregrounded "the private experience of women" (Noddings 1992, 303)— the whole school was centered around teaching, formally and informally, what a woman needs to know to keep her own mind and body and her children's minds and bodies healthy. Both the hidden and the overt curricula answered the ever-present question, what do I do when the baby arrives?

The school was organized, as Wanda Pillow says some schools for married, pregnant, and mothering teens are, with a vocational home economics focus (Pillow 2004, 152), teaching women to become both caring mothers and to earn money at low-paying, female-traditional jobs—it was a school that exemplified that troublesome "dual-role emphasis" that she writes of (Pillow 2004, 14), which she says tells us "more about what we think teen mothers deserve than what an equal education would look like for young mothers" (14). At the Teen Moms' Program where I worked there were no physics classes, no debate teams, no math classes beyond Algebra 1, no sports teams, no chess or drama or French or robotics clubs; instead, there were classes in bookkeeping, prenatal care, typing, cooking, parenting, and child development. More "safe haven" than "real-world microcosm" (Kelly 2000, 121), the Teen Moms' Program was a homey place: On cold days there was cocoa in one teacher's room, and sometimes carols around her piano; other rooms had plants on the windowsills and bean bag cushions in the corners, mobiles and children's bright purple-and-yellow finger paintings taped on the walls, and, in some rooms, bookshelves cluttered with secondhand copies of *Your Child's Self Esteem*, *Children: The Challenge*, and *Writing as a Thinking Process*. Twice a month, experts from the community came in to lecture: to show a video about how to give birth at home or to explain how to wash clothes correctly; to perform role-plays showing how to argue fairly with your husband or to describe the domestic violence shelter; to teach how to talk comfortably about sex or how to write a résumé. There were rugs on all the floors at the Teen Moms' Program, so that babies didn't skin their knees, and there was constant conversation: How had one teacher raised six children on the small salary she and her husband provided? How did another negotiate her strong career focus with her husband? Why was a third teacher still single, and how did she deal with the men she met? In many ways the school provided much more than the Thomas Jefferson and Alyssa Learning Centers did—a nurse who visited every other week, other teen moms to talk to, classes on subjects of immediate importance and a daycare center so the students could have respite from caretaking and their children could learn important skills. On the other hand, the school showed at least one of the aspects of female-only schools that research has shown to be problematic: it received fewer resources, including money and equipment (Lee, quoted in Ruhlman 1996), than such a school would have if boys studied there, too. Additionally, as Luttrell (2003) suggests, programs that "tend to target one segment of students . . . can serve to re-stigmatize those who enroll" (20). In some ways, then, the Thomas Jefferson and Alyssa Learning Centers— which worked under what Kelly (2000, 121) calls a "real-world-microcosm" philosophy, and provided traditional coursework for students of any kind who chose to go there, but no daycare center; closer connections to a community college and more individualized attention, but no classes in prenatal care, and the ability to schedule classes to suit teen mothers' busy schedules—was a better place for pregnant and mothering teens to become educated.

Wandering through the halls of the Alyssa and Thomas Jefferson Learning Centers, looking in their book rooms—stacks of paperback *Flowers for Algernon* and *The Sun Also Rises*—sitting in on classes, and in Beth's glassed-in office— "Why turn a perfectly good frog into a prince?" a sign on her bulletin board said—watching Melinda as she worked on her computer, asking questions about the students I met at the Alyssa Center—I wondered about the kind of education Gabriel, Casey, Brenda, Angel, and the other young women I saw there received.

Gabriel, Casey, Brenda, and Angel had all gone to and dropped out from traditional high schools before they became pregnant, and before they found their ways to the learning centers. I wondered what their experiences before, during, and after their pregnancies, in both the traditional and the alternative schools, were like; I wondered how being a pregnant teen in school now was different from what it had been like twenty years ago. At the Teen Moms' Program, very few of the young mothers had been from the middle class (I remembered one girl who had been a cheerleader, and the daughter of a judge): Was the experience of being pregnant in school different for middle-class students than it was for the daughters of the working-poor I'd gotten to know?

During the fall and spring of 2004 I conducted a series of interviews with women who were or had been mothers in their teenage years. Over coffee at the mall, at the library, and on the phone I spoke for four hours each with Beth Manning and Jennifer Bowles, two middle-aged, middle-class women who had become pregnant when they were teenagers many years ago; I also spoke with a woman I'll call Winnie Jones, a middle-class young mother who was making her way through the halls of a traditional high school. After the Teen Moms' Book Club disbanded, Gabriel, Brenda, Angel, and Casey met with me occasionally to talk about their experiences as pregnant teens and mothers in both the traditional schools they had dropped out from and the learning centers where I had met them.

All of the women spoke about more than their school experiences. Showing how body and mind, emotion and intellect, physical and familial context all weave together to create a young person's world, these women described parental reactions to their early pregnancies, their own longings, and their regrets. For so long in this book I have been writing about my reactions to these young women, and how the various threads of talk and image out in society frame their, and our, experiences of them. My aim in this chapter is to let the women speak for themselves.

Older middle-class teen mothers

Beth Manning: "The whole nine yards"

Over the time of my researching and writing this book Beth Manning and I had gotten to know each other well. One day we met in a conference room at the local library—a favorite haunt of ours—so that she could tell me a story I had never heard from her, about being a pregnant teen in high school. I turned on the tape recorder and Beth talked.

> I had my son when I had just turned 18 and had to get married, that's what you had to do back then (rueful laugh), in '69. Got married right away, had a big wedding, a white dress, the whole nine yards. That was no fun, no fun at all.

Beth had been raised in a lower-middle-class family in which reading and the arts were highly valued. Her family could not easily be placed by socioeconomic status, Beth thought, because her parents had values that might be associated with the upper class, in that they read classical literature and listened to the opera, but her engineer father's income might be associated more with the income of the working class. Beth was a good student and enjoyed school, but she was also "a little wild." She became pregnant, she said, not for any complex psychological reason, but because she "wasn't smart about birth control and messed around with my college-age boyfriend." Because she married when she was three months pregnant, in the April of her senior year immediately after she and her parents "found out that the reason I was so sick was because I was pregnant," and because her son was not born until she was out of high school, graduation was not difficult for her. She did not feel judged by teachers or fellow students because "it was far enough into the sixties, this was a pretty big city, and things were getting looser. It was just on the cusp of getting looser."

> Anyway. I flipped out when I found out that I was going to have a baby. For a while they couldn't figure out what was going on with me because I had a period. I was honest to the gynecologist; I said I don't *think* I'm pregnant! But . . . my dad was conceived out of wedlock, too. So my dad came into the hospital room with my mom, and the first words out of his mouth—and he was not a demonstrative man—his first words were, well let's go home and plan for the future! And my parents really were the ones who made having a baby that young and trying to raise a child be something wonderful and not something horrible, truly. And it was a mistake that did my father a lot of good because he was a heavy drinker and he'd been sober for about two years and then he'd started drinking again. And having this wonderful grandson he could be so close to—and he was very close to my son until he died—brought life back to him, it really did, it really did. They were good buddies. All three of them were very close. And I'm glad because I sure as hell didn't know what to do.

Beth's husband's parents "weren't real happy about my having a baby, no." In addition, Beth said, because she came from the "wrong side of town," she wasn't the kind of girl her husband's upper-middle-class ("pretentious") family had wanted their son to be involved with. They were angry as well when Beth's husband dropped out of college to try to support his new family. Her husband's parents didn't help them "one little bit," but her own parents supported them financially—"and we needed a lot of help!"

"That wasn't a marriage that lasted very long, and then I was a single parent for eleven years," Beth said. During those years she raised her son, finished her undergraduate degree, and began her professional career. "Those years weren't bleak. I had this little guy and he was great," she said. "We were a good team, and I had a lot of support. The only frustration was the economic part of being a single mom, and dealing with the Byzantine social services system." Beth remembers:

> Getting by on puny bits of child support and driving a car that was held together by wire. I worked full time—I worked at a trucking company for a while, and then I'd go to community college for a semester, and then I'd get another job. I'd have a roommate for a while or my son and I would live with my parents. My son would be in day care for a while or he'd go stay with his dad sometimes or my parents would take care of him. Kind of make-do. Like a lot of the kids at Thomas Jefferson. Just trying to have a life.

Jennifer Bowles: "You know I probably had a pretty good experience in my high school"

Unlike Beth, Jennifer—a forty-two-year-old wife, mother, and professional interior designer—had her son early in her high school years. Jennifer said that when she was fifteen and became pregnant out of wedlock, her father was a "main street businessman in a town of like—500," the town in which she still lives. A good student, school had always been a pleasant place for her; even the period during which she went to school pregnant she did not describe as difficult.

Jennifer linked her pregnancy to the sense of loss she felt when her grandmother died:

> Our whole household had gone through this sense of well, there really isn't anybody, 'cause my grandmother was always there, every morning when we woke up and every afternoon when we came home. My mother worked, and my grandmother, she sent us off to school. So when she died it was a sense of—oh well nobody's watching us. Part of the reason I did all that was I wanted somebody to realize that, yeah, me and my sisters were still there. It was totally—it was a total disaster. And I was having intercourse with more than one person. The sense of that whole thing was so bizarre . . . But when I got pregnant it stopped the madness I was in . . . totally stopped it.

Jennifer thought, looking back on it, that going to school as a pregnant teen was probably easier for her than it was for other girls because she lived in such a small town where "everyone knew everything about everyone." Everybody in her school had known her for a long time, and had many different visions of her identity in addition to the identity she had as a pregnant teenager. She recalled sometimes feeling that people were whispering behind her back, and she said that "still to this day" she could sometimes sense people in town pointing her out as

> that one that had the baby. But I never felt that anyone didn't like me or that—I mean

I had some friends whose parents—I think their parents chose not to let them be my friend after I got pregnant—but I had a couple of really close friends that I just stuck by. I think it was harder for the adults, when I was pregnant, because at that point it just wasn't an acceptable thing. But my friends, they understood, they were having sex with their boyfriends, too, some of them. I think it was easier for the kids than for the adults . . . and I remember a teacher—I went to school the day I was due, it was like, the 27th of August, and my home ec teacher said, when are you going to have that baby? And I was just like really big, and I said, well my due date is today, and she said, 'well, what are you *doing* here?' And she told me to go home, and I was just like, uh!

But in general, Jennifer said, her teachers had been great. Just after her son was born, she stayed home for three or four months:

The teachers from my high school came to my house. Even my biology teacher came to my house which I never ever thought he would of done, just because he was a real stern person and real judgmental, a real Dutch master, but you know what? He was probably the best teacher that I ever had. He just came and gave me all my lessons and everything. I think he even gave me a test when I was at home. He came to my house and sat with me while I took this test and to tell you the truth, I still, I was amazed. And I think every one of my teachers did visit my house. And that was great. But school went okay. I went to school like half days all the rest of high school.

Jennifer thought that being taught at home, as she was, would be the best solution for young women who have children and are trying to finish high school. She thought the idea of having a separate school for teen mothers was a terrible one:

I probably would have quit school, because that would have made me feel like they were putting me somewhere. Like, oh yeah, we'll just put her here. And I know that wouldn't have been the right thing to do either but. . . I just don't think kids should be put in a position where, you know, well, you're a bad kid and you're a good kid. You need to go to the bad school and you need to just stay in the regular school.

Jennifer had only one complaint about her schooling experience, and she made her complaint poignantly:

The only thing was when I was when I got out of high school I didn't really know what I wanted to do. I didn't have anyone really help me. Tell me what I should do and how I should go about doing it. My son was 3 when I graduated and I ended up going to a technical school and that was fine. I studied horticulture and I studied flower arranging and it was fine, but I look back on it now and think, wouldn't you want to tell someone to do whatever they want to do? They don't need to do something that's going to give them a job tomorrow—like I could of gone to college or whatever. And

I'm sure they thought, there's no way she's ever going to go to college because, y know, she's got this baby and, she could never do that, and I don't know I don't know. I mean, my life worked out okay, I have a job I really like now, but given the chance, I just don't know, I wish I had been given a chance . . .

Younger middle-class teen mothers

Winnie Jones: "It's near impossible to stay awake when you've only had two hours of sleep"

At the time I spoke with her, Winnie Jones was a senior at her high school in Bloomfield, the same little city where the Thomas Jefferson Learning Center was located. Winnie was far more supported and successful than Angel, Casey, Gabriel, or Brenda, and she was more supported and successful than most of the teen mothers described in the fiction we read in the Teen Moms' Book Club, or any of the other young-adult novels I have read about young mothers. (July Jones, of the ground breaking and problematic early novel *Mr. and Mrs. Bo Jo Jones*, is a possible exception.)

Winnie had been a star: when I spoke to her she was taking AP Calculus and AP Physics, planning on going to college in the fall to major in athletic training, and had been placed, as a gymnast, in the state finals. She was living with her parents—an engineer and an accountant—who had insisted she live with them until she graduated from high school: "They were afraid I'd move out and then I wouldn't graduate. My mom is pretty much one of the reasons I want to go to college because, she didn't. She was valedictorian of her class and she didn't go to college." Winnie seemed intent on learning from her mother's life; she seemed to have a bit of a feminist consciousness.

She worked prodigiously, going to school five hours a day and working four hours a day, at a gymnast studio in town. Her boyfriend was an older man whom she had known for a number of years; he was present at their daughter's birth. ("He's twenty-two and he works from 7–3 at Westhouser so I don't see him a whole lot. During the week. But he does the best he can and he doesn't see the baby. And that's kind of weird. My parents don't like him very much. And you know part of it is because you know he doesn't support us very much, like, at all, financially, and I don't work a whole lot so I'm—struggling.") Full of contradictions, Winnie was strong in her desire to go to college and work when she finished, but conflicted in the way she looked at her older boyfriend. I wondered whether her boyfriend could be seen in a way different from the one Winnie presented; I wondered if she was giving him more credit than he deserved.

Winnie was matter-of-fact about the work she did to keep her small family together and to move toward her goals. She spoke with assertiveness about how she worked to save money once she found out she was pregnant, about how indications from her teachers that she wouldn't finish high school only made her more determined to succeed, and about how she didn't feel uncomfortable going to school pregnant because "I guess I had enough respect for myself that I thought if they wanted to make fun of me go ahead—because it wasn't like it was on purpose—and it wasn't like everybody else isn't having sex, too, they're no different. I just got caught."

Winnie presented her experience at this traditional Midwestern high school as not being particularly difficult:

> I'm not havin' a whole lot of problems because, like, I was a really good student before, so it hasn't done a whole lot to me. One thing that I wish they could of done was when I was gone—I had her and I had to be gone and I only missed a week, yeah, I went back to school one week after having her and it was so hard for me to catch up and it was like—they were punishing me, too, the school was, and I had been punished by then, quite enough. By my parents, I mean. For five months, my parents were like, just mad at me. So it was like a struggle. And it was like I was being punished *again*. It was really hard because I'd always fall asleep because like, I start at seven, and I would fall asleep the first hour and I'd try to keep myself awake so hard but—it was—near impossible when you've only had two hours of sleep.

Winnie described both kind and unkind teachers:

> Actually—it was a guy, who was very understanding. I had my physics teacher and he was super understanding. He'd say don't worry, you can make it up in like the next three weeks, and you'll be fine. But my math teacher he was very—he told me, because it was AP math. He told me that I'd be lucky if I ever got caught up and I may have to drop his class because of it. And so—now he's like *super* good about it. It's like beforehand he was all—mean and nasty—but then he saw I was *willing* to *try* to catch up, you know I'd stay after school and I'd come in—extra. So he was like, okay, she's catching up okay. I'm that kind of person that if you tell me I can't, I'll try double hard to make it—that's pretty much—a lot of it was—I *have* to do this because I'm going to show him I'm gonna catch up. I know another girl who was pregnant whose teachers were supergood to her and stuff and helped her so she could graduate early before she had her baby. But I don't know many other pregnant girls . . .

Winnie made it clear in our conversation that she had decided not to go to the teen parent group in her town, the group that Angel religiously attended. I wondered as I spoke with Winnie if her decision was wise. I also wondered how much more difficult her life would become when she moved out of her parents' house and no longer had her mother as a full-time in-house babysitter. She planned to move in with her boyfriend as soon as she graduated, and I wondered how difficult she would find that life: beginning a more intimate relationship, raising her child more fully by herself, and going to college all at the same time. Even this very supported, very grown-up, and successful teen mom would have a hard time of it, I thought.

Gabriel Banks: "A lot of teachers are very accepting of it now"

Gabriel said that she hadn't dropped out of Alyssa High School and come to the Alyssa Learning Center because she thought teachers at her original school would be unkind to her, or because she thought the work or hours at her traditional school would be too difficult for her. "A lot of teachers are very accepting of (teenage pregnancy) now," Gabriel said, "except this one teacher who was like 65 and he had classical, traditional values." Gabriel thought that older teachers in particular ("especially men") would "have a more protective view" because "they all have daughters."

Instead, Gabriel said that she was sure that once the other students at her school found out that she was pregnant they would "treat me bad. I've known a couple of girls there who had babies, and kids didn't let them alone, they were called all kinds of names." This was the same school Casey and Brenda had dropped out of; it was a school, Brenda said, where the "preppies" picked on lower-class students; an administrator confirmed that Brenda, with her working-class accent, and Gabriel, pregnant out of wedlock, might both have felt uncomfortable in that school, one that was full of "highly motivated, wealthy students." Still, while she was at that school Gabriel had learned some things, taking Parenting and Child Development classes that would be helpful to her when she had her child: "I learned that like at different developmental stages this is all they can understand"; at the Alyssa Learning Center, with its "come-and-go" program, other students didn't bother Gabriel, but no classes in subjects like Child Development or Parenting were offered.

Push-Outs, Diversity, and the Body in School

I was surprised by some aspects of my conversations with Beth and Jennifer, Winnie and Gabriel. I had expected that certainly Jennifer's experience in high school would have been different from Beth's. Beth graduated before the passing into law of Title IX, with its language forbidding schools that receive federal funding from excluding pregnant or mothering teens from regular classes. Beth's experience of school should have been different from Jennifer's, who went to high school after 1975, after Title IX was passed. Surely, I thought, since our society has become so much more open about sexuality, and since much of our society has accepted many of the discourses connected to feminism, school life for a teen mother in the twenty-first century would be much different from—better than—school life for a teen mother in the late 1960s or early 1970s. According to the statements of Beth and Jennifer, Winnie and Gabriel, though, these differences are not as clear as I had expected them to be.

In *Unfit Subjects: Educational Policy and the Teen Mother*, Wanda Pillow (2004) suggests that though de jure segregation of teen mothers in schools has been stopped by Title IX, de facto segregation continues today. In her book Pillow describes the many ways that, today, teen mothers are subtly and not-so-subtly encouraged to drop out from mainstream schools, and either stay home and have their children or leave and go to alternative schools, if any are locally available. Pillow argues for the development of explicit policies that would encourage record keeping about teenage pregnancies and would, she thinks, lessen the de facto segregation of teen mothers (97).

Three of the women in the very small sample of middle-class, white teen mothers I spoke with described having problems that Pillow suggests are common for women attempting to continue on in traditional public high schools: Jennifer was chastised, by her teacher and in front of her classmates, for being in school at a late stage of her pregnancy (what Pillow calls "berating the pregnant/parenting teen in front of her peers" [124]); Winnie was provided few if any accommodations to help her complete the work she had to make up after being out of school during recovery from giving birth (what Pillow calls "enforcing stringent attendance requirements that do not accommodate for pregnancy and childbirth" [124]); and Gabriel feared harassment from her classmates (about which Pillow writes "unless schools have policies to explicitly define such harassment as unacceptable, as a form of sexual harassment, the teen mother will not find support for attempting to handle such instances" [100]).

It could be said that all of these white, middle-class teen mothers were encouraged to silence their pregnancies, or to keep their pregnant and mothering selves separate from school (Pillow 2004, 115). It could be said that Beth hid her unwed pregnancy by getting married, that Jennifer made her pregnancy and her mothering self-invisible by being schooled at home during part of her pregnancy, and by going to school only half days during the rest of her time in school. These two older women didn't present their experiences as being ones of hiding, however, and Jennifer clearly appreciated her teachers' kindness and help; she said that by being schooled at home she had gotten "the attention I needed." Interestingly, though, Jennifer said that her teachers and the community in general reacted more negatively to her after she had her son and decided to keep and raise him: "It was like—ooh, she *kept the baby*! Ooh, *unwed mother*!" After the baby was born, I infer, it was more difficult for school workers and community members to ignore Jennifer's choices, to ignore the fact that she was a mother, and therefore different from a traditional high school student.

Both Jennifer, in the 1970s, and Winnie, thirty years later, were expected to silence their mothering selves—Jennifer by giving her child up for adoption; Winnie by presenting a body that no longer reminded anyone that she had a child. Winnie said:

> It used to be that some teachers wouldn't give me the time of day—like I made them uncomfortable because I was different but now it's like—they don't care so much anymore, because they don't—see it anymore, I mean, they know it's there, in the back of their minds they know, oh she has a kid, but outwardly, they don't *see*—

Nathan Smith, a lean, gray-haired science teacher in blue jeans, taught at the most well-known alternative school, Circle, in Bloomfield, where Winnie lived; Circle was a school for both male and female students, but it provided special classes for teen mothers as well as an on-site daycare center. In an interview with me Nathan said that he thought some of the pregnant students who came to his school had been shoved out of the more traditional schools they had gone to. He thought both that Circle was a much better, accepting place for girls who were pregnant than the traditional school had been and that "there was a real push that Circle would be a better place for them . . . some of it would be direct but it was by and large subtle things" that teachers and administrators said and did to make pregnant and mothering students feel they would be better off at the alternative school.

> I know that although they probably already didn't fit in with peers—the stereotypic jock preppie world that the conventional school has as part of it—I don't think it's exclusively that way but that is part of it.

Nathan thought that part of the reason his students who were pregnant or mothers were encouraged to go to Circle High School was because the students were perceived as being different from most of the students in the school: it was a question of the traditional school's lack of tolerance for diversity.

In her article, "Exposed Methodology: The Body as Deconstructive Practice," Wanda Pillow (2000) frames this discomfort with diversity in another way. She suggests that school workers are uncomfortable with the teen's pregnant body—an attitude, Pillow suggests, evident today and even in schools designed expressly for pregnant teenagers. Pillow explains how the pregnant teenager's body makes adults uncomfortable because it "confounds and conflates our social norms" and "interrupts accepted and assumed demarcations of the body and self" (201). Citing popular media photographs in which the teenager's youthful face is contrasted with her swollen belly, Pillow shows how the teenager's pregnant body is openly sexual and, in schools that continue to "assume that a separation of school and body can be regulated and contained" (113), this physicality can be upsetting to school workers. Pillow describes watching girls—as Winnie probably did not—using their "challenging" bodies, bodies which brought into the schoolroom issues of pleasure and power, as "sites of resistance" in school (204). Girls who Pillow watched were clearly aware of the power that their bodies gave them. That pregnant girls suddenly have this power must be confusing for the adults they work with; it must be confusing for the pregnant girls as well. Young women who combine in their bodies the outrageousness of their youth with swollen bellies may unsettle in part because their bodies defy that "split between autonomy and sexuality" that Jessica Benjamin (1988) says "is so visible in the lives and politics of women today" (99). Citing Jane Lazarre's (1980) autobiographical writing about the connection between autonomy and a "fear of certain kinds of love" (89), Benjamin describes a desire which "often pulls women toward surrender and self-denial"; rejecting that desire in order to achieve and argue for more autonomous lives for women has caused one strand of feminism to seem "puritanical," not allowing women—especially "desexualized" mothers—to own their own complicated desire (Benjamin 1988, 91). By so clearly having succumbed to a desire that seems to be against their own self-interest, by so clearly devaluing autonomy as it is defined in middle-class, feminist thought, and by in their bodies manifesting contradictory and hard-to-settle questions about dependency, power, youth, and desire, young mothers in schools may present female school workers with discomforting personal issues they'd rather not own up to.

Working-Class Teen Mothers and School

Though the bodies of poor girls who are pregnant and mothering unsettle in the ways outlined above, I've separated out by class three young women the reader has met before. The school stories of Casey, Angel, and Brenda raise questions about school life that are different from those raised by the stories of Beth and Jennifer, Winnie and Gabriel. Contrary to what we often think, none of the working-class young women had dropped out of school *because* they were pregnant. They had all dropped out and then become pregnant during a period when they were not in school.

Casey: "I'm not kicked out, I'm done, I'm leaving, goodbye!"

It's surprising, and admirable, that Casey, Angel, and Brenda came back to school, especially given the difficult times they described. Casey and Brenda had both gone to Alyssa High School. Casey said that, during her three years there, the only good experience she had was in

> Mrs. Campbell's, the counselor's, office. We'd go out to lunch because I'd get anxiety attacks in class when I was around too many other people. When I'd freak out I'd go to her office and sit there and do art. She had this whole line of my pictures and drawings in her office; she called it 'Casey's Place.' But I dropped out when I was fifteen. People didn't like me because they thought the guy I was living with was a drug dealer but he wasn't. But I got into fights. I got into this fight with this girl, I beat her up, but after I beat her up I tried to be nice, I asked her if she was all right and all that. But the vice principal came and when I saw him I just went off, I was like, whatever. Because I'd been in so many fights, the vice principal said you're out, you're done, and I was like, fine! I quit! You know, I'm not kicked out, I'm done, I'm leaving, goodbye! Yeah!

Casey said that she had always had trouble being around groups, "I mean whether they're talking about me or not I always feel like they're talking about me, I can't do it, I can't concentrate, I can't read. . . . I didn't read. I'd be rude and mean and I'd get kicked out of class so I didn't have to read out loud." Casey believed that the teachers and students never understood the motivation for this particular bad behavior—that she was acting up in class to avoid being called on to read out loud.

Brenda: "I got so sick of being harassed"

Brenda had stories similar to Casey's. She felt that at Alyssa High School:

> you're going to get a situation like Columbine. So many kids get made fun of because

they're fat, or because—I was wearing the wrong brand of shoes . . . and they really press the issue, they'll press it every day until that person's going to snap. . . . Teachers are going to have to help the kids who are made fun of. At least, if the kids go and tell because the kids do go and tell, I did several times. I told. But still the teachers didn't do nothing. When I was going to school, I fought back when kids picked on me, but I got in trouble because I was the one that hit them, but they're the ones that pushed me first, but you know they gave them like, a warning and they gave me suspension.

Brenda said she had dropped out of high school for many reasons; she said "my mom dropped me out"; she wasn't going to school when she met her husband and drove out to Las Vegas with him. But she suggested that her problems at Alyssa High School had been related in part to her troubled family life and in part to the culture of the school:

'Cause I tried I mean I enrolled in cross country when I first started there and everything, and all the preppies, no one wanted to partner up with me. I got made fun of and the teachers just ignored it, they don't care. They treated me good, but they're not there for the problems you have at school, they're only there for teaching. They just blew it off. . . . And the whole problem is, you're still at school and you're having school problems with kids at school. I needed the help of the teachers, too, the teachers AND the principal, and not just have the principal blow off the problem. If there's a fight, they should have the two kids work out the problem with no other peers around. I got so sick of being harassed by the preppies that I fought back and I got suspended in the principal's office. Every day I had to come to school and go straight to the principal's office. By rights I do see my fault in it for pushing the student but the other student was part of it because they pushed me and I just pushed back and in that last fight there was three against one and so they took—I still think them three should of got in-school suspension too.

Brenda spoke of the difficulty teachers and administrators have addressing the complexity of school life. Though Brenda says her teachers were kind to her, for reasons we cannot know—a blindness to the need, a sense of disempowerment, an idea that problems between students were not part of their purview—the teachers she knew did not try to protect Brenda from peers who harassed her. Brenda cited this uncontrolled peer harassment—harassment based on class prejudice—as one of the main reasons she dropped out of school before graduation.

Angel: "I did feel respected by the teachers"

Angel also had school troubles before she became pregnant. She had moved from school to school for some time; on coming to this state from Alabama, the first school she had gone to was a small one:

> I was 15, 16, that's when I moved home. I didn't like it. It's not the fact that it was a regular school or the people—the people were regular pains in the butt, I didn't get along with anybody in that town. It's a very stereotyped town and if you're not born there or come there in the early years you don't fit in. Some of the girls seemed threatened by me because I seem to get along with most of the guys. And that's when I got a reputation about being all these different names.

At that school, Angel said, there hadn't been adequate courses for her "because I've been in special ed all my life and the English they had I couldn't do it." After having "fights, family troubles, me and my mom didn't get along," Angel said, she had moved in with her boyfriend's parents and gone to his school for a while.

> I did feel respected by the teachers. I never had very many problems with the teachers there. Well except for one, my special ed teacher. . . . I haven't gone and visited her in a while but when I was actually in her class I got into a lot of trouble 'cause I'm a talker. I love to talk. Normally I'm pretty shy and stuff. So I got sent out to the hall a lot. And I have a temper. Doesn't look like it but I do have a temper. Right now (at the Alyssa Learning Center) I'm doing general math so it's pretty much like adding subtracting multiplying dividing. Right now I'm dividing by decimals. I got Bs in my last two tests.

The Good That Can Come From Having a Baby Young

Though Casey, Brenda, and Angel all had trouble in school, though they all had felt unwelcome or misunderstood or simply not taken care of skillfully enough by enough people when they were in school, all three *came back* to school *after* they gave birth to their children. Each of them said they wanted to go back to school because of their changed perspective on life—a perspective changed by giving birth. They said that they wanted to earn degrees because of their children, because of their husbands, or because their new financial responsibilities caused them to take more seriously the need to go to college and/or find well-paying work. Other researchers documenting the school lives of teen mothers (Hallman 2009; Kelly 2000; Lesko 2001; Lycke 2009; Musick 1993; Pillow 2004; Schultz 2001) have made similar discoveries: Giving birth had given each of the young women I worked with a new sense of direction and motivation.

Angel:

> Well, I wanted to be able to, like when my son goes to school, I want to be able to help
> him, not be some dumb mom who dropped out of school, and I've always wanted to
> finish school because I want to be a second grade teacher. . . . So that made me want
> to get back in school. His daddy got a GED but I want to get a diploma. So I'm, I've
> got maybe about a year and a half before I get it but I'm not worried about it. Because
> I'm going to get it no matter how long it takes me. My son kind of inspired me.

Casey:

> My goal was always to be an art therapist. . . . It's a therapist who works with kids and
> people through art. . . I mean . . . when I was at the county youth shelter they had
> a book on it. So I read it and one of the workers there had a friend that was an art
> therapist. And she flew out here to talk to us. And that's my goal. And my husband
> wants me to get a college degree. . . . He wants me to—the rules are that I go to school
> or I get a job. . . . And my brother, too, he was mad at me when I dropped out. And I
> want to be able to read to my kid.

Brenda said that when she had her first child "I stopped my wildness, I stopped
my wildness, I used to drink, like—late, and all that stuff." She was planning
to give the child she was pregnant with up for adoption because she knew she
couldn't handle a fourth child "physically, mentally, or financially." She had
talked numerous times with the couple who was adopting her child:

> They said they'd take a first-class plane ticket when I start getting my contractions. I
> said, you're not going to make it! I had my first baby in five minutes, my second one,
> it wasn't any long labor either, so since this is my fourth one, when this one goes it's
> gonna be gone. By the time they're flying over—they're coming from California—by
> the time they get to Colorado I will have done popped out the baby. . . . I said to them
> you might want to come a day ahead of time.

It may seem surprising that Brenda, Casey, and Angel's lives became better
after they had their children: The idea that there is good that can come from
having a child young and out of wedlock flies in the face of our usual ideas
about teen pregnancy. But teachers I spoke to agreed with this idea, attesting
to the maturity and force that developed in their students or clients after they
had children. Juliette Baldwin said:

> Some of my clients, if it weren't for the baby, I don't know where they'd be. Some
> would be dead, or drunk, some of them it totally changes their lives, and for many
> of them, it does, for good. Some it changes their life temporarily, until the child is 2,
> 3, 5 years old, and then they shift back, but yeah, it's multiple ones I've seen it with,
> their lives have become better. . . . The very first young mom that I worked with here
> had, oh, god, multiple issues going on in her life. She has since graduated from the

university, she actually works in a profession, and is going on to graduate school, she's married, she's now just had her fourth child though, she's . . . let's see, 26. But she's done very well academically, she's actually a colleague of mine now.

Nathan Smith, the science teacher from the alternative school Circle, reinforced Juliette's comments. Nathan said his perspective on teen parenting had changed because of his relationship with one student. When I asked him, what do you think about the problem of teen parenting, he answered, "Well, what you think of as a problem, whether you think it's a problem or not is one thing." He went on:

Y'know one thing I thought about in preparation for this meeting was, I had a student who I had for a long time from 9th grade until she graduated, and that was probably at least 5, maybe 6 years, she was an advisee of mine. During that time we had a *real* good relationship, and I would say it was very parent-daughter-like. We talked a lot very candidly about all kinds of things. . . .She has three children and she was a real eye opener to me, philosophically, because I think basically it's not a great thing for high school–aged kids to have kids. And yet the kids were a savior for this young woman. Continuing to have kids was a savior for this young woman. It opened me to recognizing that there are other ways to truth and salvation than my way. This woman, I think now she's got—it's not perfect, but I think she's got a pretty together life. She's working and going to school and she's very caring about all of those kids and—the first one provided a way for her to leave her mom and the second one provided a way for her to have that intimacy she felt she was losing with the first one. And thereby she gained the strength to stand alone as a parent and not have to be dependent on a male. They're not exactly my values but I guess I've moved to a place where I don't necessarily look down my nose at young women who make those decisions. And I think by and large they're very conscious decisions to have those children. I don't always think they're motivated by the noblest intent and I'm not even sure that this young woman was *aware* of these things that I have grown aware of over time, but I still think it (having children) served a very valuable positive purpose for our society and for her. . . . I don't know for the kids.

Beth Manning said that at the Thomas Jefferson Learning Center, the pregnant and mothering teens were the students who had the least consistent attendance. Despite the fact, then, that these young women have more motivation to go to school after they are pregnant or have children than they had prior to the existence of their children, they are at the same time taking on new and confounding responsibilities that make finishing school more difficult than it would otherwise have been. Even at schools, like the Alyssa and Thomas Jefferson Learning Centers, where students can take coursework in flexible ways, where diversity is tolerated, where middle-class values are not as entrenched as they are in many more traditional schools, for these motivated working class mothers, graduating from high school will still be a monumental feat.

One of the problems is day care.

Utah, 1980:
Nine Months Poignant

March 27

Storms out. Karen unfolded her blanket and curled up next to her baby on my floor during 2nd period. Then Polly and Janet came in, excited, saying, "The cops have come to take Erin's baby away!" Liz Rosenstein talked to police and social workers and Erin left, holding her baby, crying. Her mother had called the police to tell them that Erin was an unfit mother. Nobody in this school ever saw Erin doing anything wrong to her baby. Liz said the police know that; they know that this arrest is part of an ongoing feud between Erin and her mom.

March 29

The death and dying unit in my English class has gone pretty well. We read the last act of *Our Town*, where Emily goes back to the day of her twelfth birthday; then we visited a funeral home; now girls are writing their own funeral plans. Joelle wants to be buried with her Pink Floyd records, Polly wants "Climb Ev'ry Mountain" played, and Susan wants her eulogy to mention that she was shy. All of the girls want to be described as having been good mothers.

March 30

Wendy called in, crying, today, saying she couldn't come in because she couldn't wash her clothes—they didn't have enough money for the machines, right now.

April 4

Dainty writes in her comments on my classes that last semester child development turned out better than English. I agree. Why? Basically, it was better organized, and more varied. I had films, quizzes, and readings all mapped out. In my regular English classes—not the electives—I had trouble finding material that related to their lives, that could teach them things they wanted to know.

And yet there are beautiful moments. In English, as we're talking about dogma and what it is, Jody Riggio with a sense of realization dawning on her face, says "Hey, you know what, Cindy? I'm a heretic!"

April 6

Ginelle Jones talking on the phone, crying. Just now screaming at her two-year-old, "You shut up! Just shut up!!"

Juan Hamilton, abusive boyfriend of Katie and sixteen-year-old father of Nick, isn't allowed to see his son in private. But every day at lunchtime he saunters over from the school down the hall, and, with Holly looking on, sits on a folding chair just outside the daycare center and holds his baby for a while.

April 9

Betty Jones came back to school today. Betty, who always signed her papers "Mrs. Jones," who wrote a poem in my Love Poetry class that went: *"I love you Joe oh yes I do/even when you beat me till I'm black and blue,"* Betty with her quiet dignity. The girls all say it wasn't SIDS her baby Ezekial died of. They say Betty left him with Joe when she went out for groceries, and when she came back, Ezekial was dead.

April 15

Dainty came in to show me work they've been doing in Liz Rosenstein's class. I envy Liz her English class: she gets all the motivated kids. The girls have been researching and writing a 70-page booklet—*Bright Worlds for Women*—that lists all of the medical, educational, and employment services in the county that are helpful to women. The booklet provides information about how to write a résumé, find a good daycare center, rent an apartment, or apply for financial aid, as well as addresses, phone numbers, and information about the Utah Women's Center, the La Leche League, Dress for Success offices, National Organization for Women offices, and other businesses of importance to women. The girls did all the research and writing themselves, as well as the formatting and photography for the booklet. Maybe someday I'll be as imaginative a teacher as Liz.

April 16

Word has it that Ginelle Jones's two-year-old has been taken from her. Holly from the daycare center says, "good."

April 20

Lesson plan on famous mothers

General Objectives: I have chosen four famous women, two white and two black, all of whom had children out of wedlock early in their careers. Each woman is a distinct individual with different reasons for having the baby and different reactions to having the baby. These women were chosen not so much because they were famous but because they are courageous, honest, articulate human beings who have gained a sense of their own self-worth despite obstacles. All have compassion, ambition, and humor about themselves and their lives. In short, they are all good role models for anyone--but especially for young women with babies. Hopefully, reading about these women can help my students understand themselves, see a wider range of possibilities for their lives, and gain a sense of self- esteem.

As part of this unit, I'm having the girls read the last chapter of *I Know Why the Caged Bird Sings*—the chapter in which Maya gets pregnant and has her baby boy, and "Don't Have a Baby Until You Read This," Nikki Giovanni's funny essay from her book *Gemini*; I'm also using articles about Ingrid Bergman's birth of her daughter out of wedlock—some of the articles are just scathing, attacking her morality. Maybe I could have the girls rewrite some of those articles so the tone is more positive.

When I passed out the chapter from *Caged Bird*, Tyra said, "Of course it would be a *black* unwed mother we'd be reading about." I didn't know what to say about that. Felt guilty.

April 21

Study Guide on **Caged Bird**

1. *What's a hermaphrodite?*
2. *Look up uvula in* **Our Bodies Our Selves** *or in the dictionary and be able to tell what it is.*
3. *Why did Maya have sex with the "handsome brother"? Did she enjoy it?*

Tyra and Dainty both asked me where they could find copies of the whole book. I loaned them the copy I'd got, told them where the library was. Not one girl turned her study guide in.

April 26

In English class, as part of the Famous Mothers unit, asked the girls to think of a woman they know and write down her three most admirable qualities. Tyra said, "I don't admire *women!* I admire *men!*"

May 1

Famous mothers end-of- unit test

1. *What, if anything, did each woman gain at the birth of her child? How were the women's reactions to their babies' births different? Did any woman feel negative toward her child? Why or why not?*
2. *Briefly describe each of these women's relations to the father of their children, if you can. Were they good relationships or not? Explain what you think a "good" relationship is.*
3. *Explain what qualities each of these women have which you admire, if there are any.*

May 13

Cream-colored roses on the railing outside my apartment. Pulling pink and purple finger paintings down from the windows of my classroom, unpinning "A" papers from the bulletin board, dropping my file folders into boxes. How the room got less empty as the year went on! Told Dainty and Tyra of the sweet smile about their grades. Dainty got an A- in English and Tyra got a B. "Hey, you must think she better than I am," said Tyra. Smiling, swinging out the door, she said, "I'm going ta git you for that, Cindy."

May 15

Tonight, under my great-grandmother's quilt in my lumpy Murphy bed, I can't sleep. I don't know if it's all the coffee or all the thoughts curling through my brain. Tonight the Teen Moms' Program had its banquet honoring the graduating seniors. I walked alone in my fancy new sandals and my grown-up teacher dress, past blue mountains and lilac just nose-level to the Front Room, a glittering downtown restaurant. It was all education talk and the seniors with tears dripping from their mascara, wearing high heels and backless dresses, eating roast beef and potatoes at long white cloth-covered tables with their husbands and boyfriends and parents. When the awards ceremony started, the building principal introduced me as the only member of the staff who was still single.

Every senior received an award: for kindest, most dedicated student, most improved. Joyce and Tyra handed each teacher a bunch of yellow-ribboned daisies. They gave a special bouquet to Holly from the daycare center, and started crying, almost in unison. "Thank you for—Holly Jenson—for being patient and for teaching us so much." Big Carmen hugged me and gave me a "special thanks" because I'd "meant so much to her." What a surprise!

May 17

I feel like a graduating senior myself, I feel nine months poignant. Last night Liz and I went to the Adult Ed graduation, to see our seniors march across the stage. The commencement speaker gave a talk called "Nonpositive Thinking or How to Succeed and Fail at the Same Time." You never know what you don't know until you try it and find out what you don't know and then it's called a failure. An eighty-year-old man graduated and as one woman walked across the stage someone yelled out, "Way to go, Mom!" A man in blue jeans and an untucked plaid shirt whooped when he came down the stairs. After she received her diploma a woman my mom's age just stood very quietly and cried, wiping her hands on her skirt. And from the Teen Moms' Program, Rosie and Maria and Tyra and Polly and Dainty and Susan.

In my classroom Sandy asked anxiously, "You'll be here on Tuesday?" And Maria and Polly, about to go to community college, melancholy about moving into a new phase. At lunch the old teacher Ladene Welker in her checked pants, licking the blue cheese dressing off her fingers, saying to Liz Rosenstein, "You know, Liz, I really worry about these girls. What will happen to them?"

Chapter 7

These Kids Are Starved for Knowledge

Because I was so focused on learning how to run my classroom I wasn't aware, when I taught at the Teen Moms' Program, of how important the one-room daycare center was. I saw the children of students marching down the hall in Batman capes with Holly, the daycare center director, shouting, "We're macho kids!" and I saw babies rocking in cribs when I visited the bright daycare room. I knew that some of my students took turns working with the children and babies who stayed in the daycare center while other girls were in classes and I saw how much my students appreciated Holly's work. Some students knew they needed to educate me: A girl explained how grateful she was that her daughter was in school with her because, "Look," she said, staring down at her chest, "my milk runs whenever I hear a baby cry. It hurts. But here, when that happens, I can just walk across the hall and see how Oscar's doing."

But not being a mother myself yet, none of this really sunk in, back thirty years ago. When, during the fall and spring semesters of 2004, I spoke with teachers and counselors and teen mothers, in coffeeshops and libraries, classrooms and parks, on the phone and in person, I heard the strong cases they made for housing daycare centers within school buildings, and for defining differently a school's relationship to community services. I spoke with teachers and counselors Jenny Moore, Letitia Moss, Nathan Smith, Melinda Vane, Carol Johnson, Beth Manning, and Juliette Baldwin—for about 30 hours of both formally structured and more informal interviews; I went back often with follow-up questions. These teachers and counselors described benefits I hadn't thought of; they spoke of the good learning a daycare center provides all students in a school community.

In addition to discussions of the promise and problems associated with centering daycare in school buildings, these teachers and counselors argued for schools that were full service in other ways, describing the benefits—particularly to working-class and poor students—of having a nurse and social worker at a school site full time. They also talked about how, in their classrooms, they tried to balance student-focus and content-focus, care and rigor: they argued for new ways of thinking about what it means to succeed in school. They described the sadness they'd experienced when they taught teen mothers; they described the qualities of character and education they thought teachers of students, who are considered educationally out of the mainstream, might need.

Flourish Is the Word

"Sometimes when I drop Ben off at his daddy's," Angel said one afternoon as I was getting into my car to make the drive home, "he's clinging to my shirt."

> It's like he doesn't want to go, it's like he doesn't want to see his daddy. Like he's scared of his daddy. I know Jason gets—impatient with having Ben over there sometimes. Jason's got a real bad temper . . .

I worried about Angel and her son Ben when I was at work, when I was driving to the Alyssa Learning Center, and when I was at home with my own son. I remembered how much the director of my son's daycare center had helped me when I had worries, or needed to be taught something about childrearing, and I thought about how isolated Angel seemed, despite her connection to the group that helped young parents. Was Ben just showing typical symptoms of separation anxiety, which Angel didn't recognize, being new to mothering? How much did Angel really know about how Jason was treating Ben? How could she find out? I thought about Rachel at the Teen Moms' Program, who had left her husband not because he hit her, but because she couldn't stand to think that he might hit their child. I had spoken with Melinda Vane about Angel's sometimes-violent relationship with Jason, and Melinda had said that she, and the school—where Angel was only sometimes enrolled—had no authority to help Angel since she had withdrawn domestic abuse charges against Jason.

Juliette Baldwin, the young woman who ran the Youth Services Program for teen parents, told me that Angel's situation—her fear that her child's father, an essential family caretaker, might hurt her son—was not unusual. If Angel had been able to find a school that had a daycare center attached to it, Juliette suggested, she would have been free from this kind of worry. But since the Welfare Reform Act of 1996 and its reinstatement in 2002, Juliette said,

> We've seen that teens no longer qualify for welfare and they're forced to stay at home with their parents and in some cases that's been beneficial but in other cases that hasn't been beneficial because there is substance use, drugs, and violence in the home and kids are forced to stay there with their children where they'd be better off on their own.

Letitia Moss, a lively Southerner and PhD candidate in education, introduced herself to me one day in a class; she had heard that I was working with teen mothers, she said, and wondered how she could help. Later she told me that her twenty-year career had been exclusively centered on working as a counselor, tutor, and parenting class teacher of pregnant and mothering teens at traditional high schools and pregnant teen centers in Ohio and the Carolinas. We met one day in front of the local library and made our way through slush to a conference room where we could talk. Did any of the schools where she taught have daycare centers, I asked Letitia eventually, and did she think that had been beneficial to her students? Letitia settled herself into the chair across from me and talked carefully into the tape recorder:

> Now, it depended where I was at. When I was at the one school—career and technical education school or vocational school I guess you might say—we had a child care program. We had a nursery school and we had an infant care program as part of it. And so the teens would bring their children with them to school and then during their lunch they'd spend it with their child and then after school they'd be there, too. And it was really nice. We noticed their attendance rate went way up because they brought their child with them. However of course it was looked at differently by different people, like "well let's just make it easy fer them, let 'em all git pregnant, we're gonna take care a their kids too." You know this is the way the argument would go. But I saw the beauty and—the flourishing of the relationship between the mother and the child and also the benefit of watching what other parents did when they took care of the kids, and also of just having a break.
>
> I remember one girl, her baby—let's say her baby was named Suzie—and Suzie it was obvious, didn't have stimulation, I mean nothing. You know children track, do this (Letitia held up her finger and followed it with her eyes as she moved it back and forth) automatically, most children do tracking automatically. With Suzie, there was no tracking. She'd look straight ahead. She had had no stimulation but—(Letitia whispered in wonderment) I watched this child—well, *flourish* is the word. And the more she was worked with at school and plus the mother was working with her and taking an interest, and this baby just flourished.
>
> However, the bad side is that after they had been at the school for two or three years a new principal came in—female, to boot—you'd think she'd be for it but she said I don't want any of that in my school! She came from a school where no one gets pregnant. So that was the end of the care center.

I remembered how Juliette Baldwin described the daycare at the Youth Services Center where she worked. She and Letitia highlighted the same benefits. The picture she created, however, suggests how costly, in terms of staff, a really well-put-together daycare center might be:

The intention of the daycare at the Youth Services Center is twofold: one intention is to reduce the incidents of child abuse among children of teen parents who are at much higher risk than non-teen parents for committing abuse. And the other intention is to provide an opportunity to give the child stimulating play. It's very structured, we only take 4–5 children and we generally have at least 3 staff so it's almost one-on-one attention, so we can assess the child developmentally and work on stimulating that child because children of teen parents are much more likely to lag behind developmentally and are twice as likely to repeat a grade once they're in school . . . so the daycare is our way of doing early intervention services with the kids.

Nathan Smith, the thoughtful, gray-haired, blue-jeaned science teacher we have met before, had taught at a variety of alternative schools. He had taught at a school I'll call Horizon before he moved to the alternative school where he presently taught, Circle. Both schools had students who were pregnant or mothering as well as students who were male or not mothering; both schools housed daycare centers. Nathan described some of the benefits these centers provided for all of the students at the schools:

Horizon had associated *intimately* with it a daycare and so although not *every* parent used that daycare, most did, and that provided all kinds of wonderful things. I mean, you know, whether it be access between parent and the child—if the kid's fussy or whatever—the parent could go down there—to modeling good parenting skills and childrearing techniques, to a kind of a support group of other young women who were in the same situation. I think it really provides a venue for boys to be a little more nurturing than they get to be at that age at a high school, too. At Circle there's a lot of taking care of these young pregnant moms by boys who are not significant others in these girls' life. Yeah, it's kind of positive. I think both of those places (Circle and Horizon) provided opportunities for non-parenting students to work in the daycare, and for some of them it served as a legitimate substitute for them—I mean a substitute for having their own children—and I don't know intimately of *anyone*—I know first hand of no student whose experience there led them to become a parent, but I do think it may have dissuaded some students from becoming parents, or made them think about it twice . . .

It's interesting that both Nathan and Letitia mention counterarguments to having daycare centers in high school buildings—the fear that somehow daycare in the school building might encourage teens to have children. Both Nathan and Letitia suggest that, in their experience, this fear is unfounded.

Winnie Jones, the middle-class young mother I described in the last chapter, had a different concern. When I asked her what she thought about having a daycare center attached to a high school, she responded with a description of the center at Circle, the alternative school described above, that was very different from the rosy picture Nathan painted:

> The only problem with the daycare at Circle is, I know a guy that worked in the daycare there and he was the scariest person I've ever met in my whole life. It'd be like kids taking the class and working in the daycare because daycare's an easy class. They spend an hour there and it's like oh! All I have to do is watch the kid get into trouble and I get credit for it! Circle's a school for kids that don't want go to school and don't want to try but they want to get their GED.

It's difficult to know if Winnie's ideas came from a prejudice against Circle and the kinds of students who matriculated there—like many middle-class, white, college-bound students she saw the school as a kind of dumping ground, calling it a "black" school—or if her comments described a situation that others might also see as a problem. Nathan told me that teachers at daycare centers, by law, had to be certified to teach; he said that the woman who supervised the daycare center at Circle was the mother of children herself, was certified as a nurse as well as a teacher, and had been the director of the center for many years. Letitia's comments about the female principal who shut down the daycare center speak to questions about where administrators put their priorities, and the money at their disposal, when they educate students. Certainly daycare centers housed in schools would need to provide strict, educated, caring, and competent supervision both of the children being cared for and of the teenagers who work with them.

Winnie Jones and Jennifer Barnes, predictably, had fewer problems finding good care for their children than the working-class young women I interviewed did, because they had fewer economic constraints. Still, there were problems the middle-class women experienced that having a daycare center in or near their schools might have alleviated. Here's what Winnie had to say when I asked her where her daughter stayed when she was at school:

> When I'm at school she goes to a lady that used to work at Kiddie Care—she was going to teach and then they had a oops I got pregnant. And she's like, twenty four, and she has a child that's three, and she's like, oh I have a baby now I want to stay home with my baby. I think it's good for my daughter to be around her son, I think that's good for her because she needs some social interaction, she doesn't see that many people I mean she's there, and then we come home and she's with grandma and then we spend a little time together when I get home, and she doesn't really see that many people in the day.

> Sometimes I miss her when I'm at school and sometimes it's a relief. Oh, all right, I get to be normal for a little bit. Sometimes also like my mom'll watch her at night on the weekends and that's also—like, I miss her up to a point but it's also like hey I get

to be normal for like, 3 hours, and I'm like, I'm not, a mom. And sometimes it's like I wish I could go out and do somethin' and I just can't because I have to be here with her and that's hard because people want me to do stuff without her too and I can't. Friends of mine, they're like, hey you wanna? And I'm like, nope! Probably no-ot . . . And it's hard for them to understand how I care about her like you don't understand what being a parent is like until you *are* a parent.

Winnie said, "It feels like, it may be really common or it may be totally off the wall but it feels like I'm not really raising her, like my parents are just raising another child." Jennifer's mother also took care of the baby while Jennifer was going to school; Jennifer said that

the hardest part [of having a baby young] for me was that my mom was the mom and I always felt like she was making all the decisions . . . like my son was really hers. I wanted to decide but I didn't want to decide, too. I was very—I'd just go away, be gone, leave. I'd stay at my boyfriend's house for a couple of days and my parents would call me and say, you cannot do this, you have to come home.

This conflict between generations is a quite typical problem for teen parents. The conflict between the teen mother's need to be a teen—hanging out with her friends and boyfriend, rebelling against her parents—and her need to be self-abnegating as a mother is common as well. Juliette Baldwin explained this aspect of teen parenting:

We would like to see kids complete the stage of adolescence right now, when they're supposed to, although that's in strong contrast to being a good parent. You know we think of adolescence as being a time to explore your identity. Kids are impulsive, they're self-focused, and those qualities don't jibe with being a responsible parent.

According to these women, then, having a daycare center housed in a school building could help both working-class and middle-class adolescent mothers have time to "be normal for a little bit" and might alleviate some intergenerational conflicts as well.

Juliette told me that the district-wide daycare centers in her town, available to teen parents going to traditional schools as well as to teen parents going to the alternative school, were vastly underfunded:

This year the school district daycare center's been overwhelmed. Presently there are 17 girls on the waiting list and I know that some of those girls have been unable to go to school. Also daycare funding is a problem—there's a huge waiting list for state-funded daycare and unless you're receiving welfare benefits you don't get on a waiting list. A majority of our folks don't qualify for welfare because they are under 18. So they have to be placed on a waiting list for the school district daycare and no one has moved off that waiting list this year. So that's created a problem—some girls have been forced to drop out of school or find substandard daycare, which puts children at great risk.

We just had a little four month old whose leg was—he had a bone fracture because he was left in substandard care and this was a mom who was on a waiting list for the Learning Place daycare and now the child is in foster care. So one wonders if there hadn't been that long waiting list and that child had been in a quality center, that child probably wouldn't be in foster care right now.

Juliette made these statements more than seven years ago; I wonder how much more overwhelmed such care centers are now, when so much energy and money is still focused—despite our new president—on making sure students do well on state and national tests.

Here They Can Get Two Critical Things at the Same Time

All of the adults I spoke with wanted more than just daycare centers in or near the schools where teen mothers studied; they wanted schools that were "fullservice" in other ways as well. In *Full Service Schools: A Revolution in Health and Social Services for Children, Youth, and Families*, independent researcher and writer Joy G. Dryfoos (1994) writes about how important it is to combine "the settlement house with the school" (12), especially for poor students; she describes the long history of this conception: the idea of bringing health and social services into the school began as early as 1890, with Jane Addams and the entry of immigrants to school (21). Dryfoos shows how the idea of the full-service school has been more or less well received, depending on which political party is in power in the White House. Dryfoos lists the many prospering full-service schools available in 1994 and the data that describes the benefits such schools confer on their students. Warning that "the difficulties of evaluating multicomponent programs have been fully documented" (123) and suggesting that more research is needed, she describes lowering of drop out, early pregnancy, and substance abuse rates associated with providing health services, including daycare, in the schools. She highlights one school in particular, IS 218 in Washington Heights, New York, which joined with the Children's Aid Society to create a school in which there are dance classes and breakfast at 7 a.m., a wide variety of choices for educative after-school programs from 3 – 6 p.m., a family resource center that helps with immigration and citizenship issues, public assistance, housing, crisis intervention, and adult education; a clinic to which parents and children can come for dental visits, well-child visits, and prenatal care; a small mental health center, and a daycare center (100–108). She describes how the community paid for the services in this school, and quotes one foundation officer who visited IS 218 asking, "How do we get this in every school?" (106).

Barbara Tye (2000), who wrote *Hard Truths: Uncovering the Deep Structure of Schooling*, and Andy Hargreaves (1997), who edited *Rethinking Educational Change with Heart and Mind*, also advocate for full-service schools. Tye calls the goal of moving toward developing full-service schools a "substantive project" and connects this change most clearly to the needs of those in the innercity. As she cautions against taking on too many changes at once, she describes the need for moving toward creating schools that are "truly the hub of [their] communities," schools that provide before-and-after school programs as well as "services ranging from dental care to night-school classes" (173). Hargreaves (1997) describes the kinds of help teachers need in order to "accommodate the multiple intelligences and varied learning styles of culturally diverse students" (7) and writes of one "more radical" solution to this new need: "the idea of locating social work and youth services in the school so that teachers and social workers can collaborate for welfare of their children" (7).

Juliette Baldwin said,

> I think there are some [of the young moms she works with] that are real reluctant to use our services and often times those are folks that have had lots of contact with the system, as they call it, growing up, and they have a strong distrust with any sort of counselor or social worker who would come into their home.

These young women in particular, it would seem, young women, perhaps, like Casey and Gabriel, whose tough exteriors and pride would make it difficult for them to ask for help, whose complicated lives would make it difficult for them to find time to visit Juliette's offices, and who instinctively mistrust the kinds of people who work there, would benefit from being able to obtain more readily in the schools some of the kinds of caring services Juliette's teen parent program provides. In a similar fashion, the middle-class student Winnie, who had decided against going to the teen parent program that Angel went to, would have been helped by having a few conversations with a social worker, were such a person easily available to her through school.

Nathan Smith suggested some of the benefits of having more services in the schools when he described the alternative school, Circle:

> Circle has a nurse practitioner on staff and she's very involved with both the parents

and the kids. I'm sure that's just an enormous boost with the routine stuff. I was thinking the other day as I was walkin' out the door there was a mom holding her kid and the nurse had her otoscope in her ear, lookin' at the kid as she was going out the door. So she's trackin' it—the baby's care—we talked about how a teen parent has a hard time getting to school, well, they have a hard time getting to the doctor, too—service is a real problem—and here, at Circle, they can get two critical things at the same time.

Not a "Real School"

As I was talking to Nathan, Letitia, and Juliette about the changes they wanted, and had seen work, from their positions slightly outside the traditional educational system—Nathan as an alternative school teacher and Letitia and Juliette as teacher-counselors connected to schools, but not always teaching traditional classes—I remembered the boys from Utah High School, whom I mentioned in Interlude 3. Those boys must have thought the Teen Moms' Program wasn't a "real school" at least in part because it contained so many of those full service functions the adults I was speaking to wanted. Perhaps the boys thought the Teen Moms' Program wasn't a "real school" also because it served what they thought of as a lowly population—girls, especially girls who've made "mistakes," girls who, being pregnant, are defined perhaps more than usual by their bodies.

If this is true, then the boys from Utah High were expressing ideas that are so normal and natural (St. Pierre 2000, 485), so widespread, as to be invisible. These ideas assume a splitting off of different aspects of human experience (Luttrell 1997, 9), and they structure the institutions in which we educate most students. Traditional high schools tend to privilege the academic part of education over the social part and school knowledge over practical knowledge (Luttrell 1997, 9). Another way of saying this is that traditional schools value representational knowledge over experiential knowledge. Generally speaking, traditional high schools also tend to valorize the side of human experience not associated with the feminine (St. Pierre 2000, 481). Most traditional high schools value rigor over care, intellect over emotion, mind over body, work over play. This overvaluing of one side of human experience is perhaps another reason that administrators and policy makers are not as open to housing social services associated with caring in the high school as the teachers I spoke with would like.

In *Moral Boundaries*, a thoughtful argument for the centrality of caring work in social and political life, Joan Tronto (1994) shows how in the United States "taking care of" is work for white men, while "caring for" activities are devalued, underpaid, and disproportionately occupied by the relatively powerless in society. In the United States, "cleaning up" jobs are disproportionately held by women and men of color (113). . . . In addition, those who are thought of as "others" in society are often thought of in bodily terms: they are described by their physical conditions, they are considered "dirty," they are considered more "natural." Thus, the ideological descriptions of "people of color" and of "women" (as if such categories existed) often stress their "natural" qualities: in dominant American culture, blacks have a sense of rhythm and women are naturally more nurturant and emotional. (114)

Teachers who work primarily with teen mothers—caregivers teaching "others" thought of "in bodily terms"—are perhaps seen as less educated, less respectable, than teachers who work in traditional schools. Because of their association with students seen in "bodily terms," these teachers may feel powerless more often than teachers who work with more mainstream students do. Certainly the teachers I interviewed thought about how the perceived splits between work and play, body and mind, emotion and intellect, played out in their lives at school. They described questions that troubled them, like: How can a student study when she's worried about her child? Which is more important, expressing intelligent care or demanding responsibility from students? How to do both at the same time? How important is it to assume an attitude of creativity and playfulness when completing serious schoolwork? In a curriculum for pregnant teens, which should be provided more space, learning how to care for the body or learning how to care for ideas?

Letitia Moss said:

> I think schools have to have a vested interest in children because they aren't perfect and if you showed the child that you care, maybe they'll feel a little bit better about themselves, and maybe that'll reflect more positively on their children. You *have* to care. There would be some teachers that would be *wonderful* with these students and there'd be others that'd be cut and dry—here are the RULES and you didn't turn this *in* at this *date* on this *time*—NO extension! I'm sorry if your child was sick, but, too bad! I saw a lot of that, oh yeah! On the other hand, I know children need to be accountable to some degree and so—(she held out her hand in a gesture expressing the complexity of the balance to be made)—caring—

Nathan Smith had a similar view about the balance an institution can keep between strictness and understanding, consistency of expectation and making allowances for individual needs:

> I think the parents at both the alternative schools that I have worked in are very much

just one of the kids. And yet there's a special role and there's accommodations made for them by both staff and their peer friends. Everybody understands that this girl may be in five minutes late to science class because she's been off to the nurse with her kid. It's no big deal, it's just part of the circumstances and the other kids are very accepting. I think that's a really nice thing about alternative schools. Everybody comes together as a group. Everybody is very tolerant of everybody's little bit weirdnesses that put them off the mainstream.

Think about how different that attitude is from the position of Winnie Jones's math teacher, who told her she might have to drop his class. In some schools, and with some teachers, being a little bit late to science class, or missing a week of class to give birth, would be seen as a lack of commitment or discipline; ensuring that discipline was kept could be seen as part of demanding rigorous attention to studies. One of the reasons it's difficult to stop the intense focus on absences, extensions, and students' "little bit of weirdnesses" is that a bookkeeping type of evidence is easier to maintain, more reliable in some ways, than evidence that students are genuinely exploring sophisticated ideas when they are in class.

These Kids Are Starved for Knowledge

This need for measurable evidence of learning must be one reason that we in secondary schools cling so tightly to the "Carnegie unit" (1995) that "academic accounting device" that consists of "a course of five periods (taken) weekly throughout an academic year" (Tyack & Cuban 1995, 91), each "period" being about fifty to fifty-five minutes long. The Carnegie unit provides us with a clear, measurable, black-and-white way of accounting for learning. Along with many others (Tyack & Cuban 1995; Tye 2000), Wells (1996) suggests that another reason the definition of rigor that ties it to the Carnegie unit is difficult to change is the common idea that "school ought to be hard; it doesn't matter if kids like it" (177). All of the alternative school teachers in this study spoke about the value of loosening the hold of the Carnegie unit on schools to allow for more flexibility for students who need to work or take care of their children. Nathan Smith, for one, made a persuasive case:

> The other thing was that the academic program at Horizon was set up to provide kids credit for work they did in *teeny* increments. And the conventional school is limited by this huge bureaucracy that forces them into giving kids credit or no credit for a whole term. Whereas for a parent, that can be a real problem. You get the kid sick, you're going to have some problems, and you're out of school for a couple of weeks. All of a sudden it's *impossible* for that parent to earn credit so they lose a whole term's worth

of credit. Well at Horizon they'd get credit for the three weeks they'd put in before
then. In fact, we had a system of carrying *every minute*, so that even if they didn't earn a
whole credit they'd get *half* a credit worth. It was kept in a *bank* by the curricular area
so when they came back later, it would roll in and they'd still get it. So I think that was
real beneficial to parents. You know with children it's real hard to have the kind of
regular attendance that the conventional high schools expect.

Though Winnie was clearly disdainful of her local alternative school,
Circle—she described it as a "scary place" where "the math classes are so easy
I could do them in my sleep"—she would have benefited from the flexibility of
credit attainment, that dislodging of the Carnegie unit, that alternative schools
have been allowed.

In a similar fashion, it's clear that Angel and Brenda benefited from the
flexibility of credit attainment available at the Alyssa and Thomas Jefferson
Learning Centers. Angel hadn't been able to go to school for some time after
her son Ben was born because she couldn't study at a full-time school, and find
care for her son:

I didn't want to go to school there because you had to go eight hours a day and I didn't
have a babysitter to take care of Ben. So finally I went down to talk to the alternative
school to find out if they had anything like this here at Alyssa and they said yeah we
have a completion class but it's only open on Tuesdays.

Brenda had been able to take classes at her own quick pace at the Thomas
Jefferson Learning Center. All of her teachers saw how hard she worked, and
encouraged her. She said,

I finished this class here in like nine days . . .but I'm already ahead of the class, so I was
thinking of asking Jody if I can not show up for the classes but come after the classes
and just take the test. That way I can get to my job. I can just take the test and finish up
this class. . . . That's one of the good things about this school, they will navigate with
you, because they navigated when I was coming to school here from like nine to two.
They would work with me, because they knew I needed to get home and sleep.

Students other than teen mothers might benefit from the dislodging of the
Carnegie unit; Beth Manning described students who did not have children
or problems that caused them to drop out of the more traditional schools, but
came to Thomas Jefferson simply because they wanted to finish more quickly
than students can in traditional schools:

We've got a bunch of high school students who felt bored, they wanted to go faster
with school or they wanted to also work, so they do all their studying at home, and

just come in and take the tests. Three of them, in fact, this week, that I was working with, working on American Government 2, they're whizzing through it. It's a very difficult class as a teacher-led class, let alone as a self-study class, and we have running jokes about them because if they dropped down to a 97% we're going, well, shoot, Lauren, what happened here? What's wrong with you? (Beth laughed) Jeff, I believe that Mariah's ahead of you . . . . They just want to live their own lives the way they want to live them. They don't like being in traditional schools, they don't, and they're really smart.

I worried, though: Can a school provide needed "rigor" if credit is attained in what Nathan Smith called "teeny increments"? What does that chopping up of study do to a student's concentration, to the depth of her understanding of the subject? Do these "teeny increments" make it more difficult for students to learn how to read increasingly dense and conceptually sophisticated texts, and to link these texts with others? How well can a school that counts credit in this more flexible way scaffold students' learning? I asked Beth Manning if she thought that, even without using the Carnegie unit to mark students' progress, students were provided a good education at the Thomas Jefferson Learning Center.

Yeah, I think students do get a good education. I think it would be better if they could do all their coursework in a classroom rather than by themselves, I really don't think that's the best fit for most of these students. I wish we had a lot more to offer, but we can't, we just don't have the budget. I wish we had all sorts of classes. I know we all wish we had a daycare center and special mom-classes. I have told some teens who move from our program to Circle that I think that's a good idea. At Circle they have on-site childcare, they've got all these wonderful classes about parenting, and they have a wonderful program there, and they've got a lot more classes than we've got here. But yeah, I think what we offer is good. It's not enough.

The kids here are starved for knowledge, any kind of knowledge. A lot of times the reason they act disinterested is because it's foreign territory, something to be afraid of, especially because they don't want to look dumb. All those defense responses could easily be misconstrued as an outward sign of a different valuing system. . . . I would say that alternative high schools and adult high schools are uneven in their approaches today. More alternatives used to be considered "soft," too much caring, not enough rigor, so to speak. Most folks currently working in alternatives have felt that what has been offered in the past was second rate, and that the rationale behind a second-rate education for these kids and adults was that they don't need that high level stuff. So, lots of schools had good nurturing and only basic education types of classes taught by whoever was around. Fortunately those underlying premises have been challenged as it became clear that what was really being offered was inferior education—separate and unequal, the outcome of which, of course, keeps these kinds of students stuck in lower paying jobs with little skills to move upward. Things have changed now, I think, and people who work in alternative schools are trying to improve the education, make it more rigorous. We're more aware of students' educational needs, too. They don't always want the same kinds of knowledge that kids in more traditional schools do, but they want to learn things about life, about how it all works. They are starved for knowledge, any kind of knowledge, and I think they can get that now.

Something to Behold

Nathan, Letitia, and Beth all spoke of the skills they had learned and the skills they thought teachers needed to use, when they were working with pregnant and mothering teens; they spoke of the emotional toll this work sometimes took. Nathan suggested that, like elementary school teachers, teachers who work with students who are as needy as some teen mothers tend to use a more child-centered pedagogy than teachers who work in more traditional high schools:

> Where I came in to alternative schools is from elementary schools because I'd gone to kind of a radical elementary teacher prep program that was very child centered. I decided that for me, even though it was very child centered, even though I wanted to teach high school science, it was the right focus. I think that's probably true of many alternative school teachers, I think many alternative school teachers focus more on the child, caring for the child, than they do on the subject. On the other hand I think alternative schools are real tough for young inexperienced teachers. I've watched a number of young teachers just be consumed by the amount of neediness and hurt and anger their students bring them. But I think we all think the kids come first.

Beth described the ways in which the Thomas Jefferson Learning Center allowed her more freedom, and required more responsibility from her, than a traditional school would.

> I really do make Thomas Jefferson a peaceful place. The students know it from the beginning, it's got to be mutual respect from everybody to everybody, it's got to be a safe place and a peaceful place. That's where I've got a lot more leeway than a regular school because I do tell people to go if they are too disruptive. Leave today and come back tomorrow but if you can't be here, you can't be here. I'm really protective of that environment and I think a lot of those teen moms are really comfortable with that. And they can be there when they need to be, not be there when they are in a bad way and just can't come. They also like the structure of the classes, they love the fact that there is zero tolerance in our classes for any kind of disruption because the teachers come to me and say I need this person out of there, and that's it, that person is gone. The teen moms really appreciate—and I really appreciate—that we can make those kinds of allowances, and those kinds of rules, at our school.

Letitia's friend and colleague Carol Jones spoke of how irritated she sometimes felt with her pregnant students, how she wanted to tell them to "study something!" since they were so often "sitting around" waiting for their boyfriends to come back.

> I see a very slight change in maturity level between the time they are pregnant and the time their children are born. When they are pregnant, they're all worried about how much it's going to hurt, but after they have their child they have to get a bit more practical, and start thinking about clothing and feeding their children. I really like helping them learn how to take care of their bodies. For some of them it's the first time they've ever been healthy, the first time they've learned about proper nutrition.

Carol sounded a little tired to me, as if she needed time away from the emotional work her students required of her. Her conversations made me think of Hargreaves's writing about how, when "the demands of caring feel overwhelming" (1065) teachers sometimes "insulate" themselves from their students, sometimes by blaming them. Hargreaves suggests that this blaming is one way teachers come to terms with their feelings of "powerlessness and helplessness" (1065).

Letitia also spoke of how difficult some of her students were. Teachers in some schools where she had worked envied her, she said, because she had such small classes. Teachers at other schools, particularly in what she called "inner-city schools" welcomed her into the building because the teens she taught were perceived as difficult:

> Especially at the beginning of their pregnancies when they didn't want anyone to know they were pregnant, they would act out a lot in class so that the teachers just hated 'em. So they really were glad I was there, to take 'em out of class and work with them.

But

> One thing that I noticed, talking about caring and now I'm talking about the teacher caring—you can only do it for so many years because it becomes very depressing. It's the same story over and over. I hate to say it's the same story, because it's not the same story but it *is*. Over and over and over, the similar dysfunctions. And just watching the bubble burst, and then in the long run the girls end up blaming the boy, and then the child, especially if the child misbehaves and they think the child is bad. And the guy disappears as soon as he hears that she's pregnant. And it's just overwhelming, watching the family situations over and over again . . .

I asked Letitia how she had managed to deal with that sorrow, that drain, for twenty years. First she said, "I just feel . . . there's nobody to speak for these girls, and I wanted to be one who did. They need so much help, and they try so hard . . ."

Letitia paused to think. She looked at me and said, "You know there's all kinds of evidence, research, that graduating from high school is one of the best things young moms can do for themselves. They tend to have a second child less often if they graduate from high school, and I think they are less prone to abuse the children. You can look that up. But me? What I did to rejuvenate myself was I never missed a graduation.

"That's how I really dealt with the repetition of the dysfunction, the wondering how much of a difference I'd made, the sad stories. I went to every graduation. I celebrated every success. I just . . . that fact that some of those girls got through, with all their problems. Lord have mercy, those girls' graduations were something to behold."

Chapter 8

Stories You Have Told Me

At the beginning of this book and throughout it in small interludes I've woven parts of a story about the year I spent teaching English and other subjects in a little alternative school for pregnant, married, and mothering teens. At the school I've called the Teen Moms' Program—just above the Youth Eager for Truth School, across from the ESL program for Vietnamese, Cambodian, and Laotian refugees, and down the hall from the school for juvenile delinquents—I first began asking some of the questions this book attempts to address. Reading novels about teen mothers in my rowdy English class, I began wondering about the difference between the young-adult novels we read and the stories my students lived. Trying to play volleyball in the mornings with the girls I've called Dainty, Rosie, and Susan, I began thinking about the conversations we might have about the complexities of living in a female body, and the confusions of desire. Teaching child development and econ and health classes from textbooks cast off by the regular high school, I began to wonder what equal education for poor women, particularly poor women with children, would look like.

I've answered, in small ways, some of the questions I started asking so many years ago. I've answered three main questions: How did the young mothers I got to know, in taking in bits of the discourses around them and rejecting others, try to construct new and more generative life stories for themselves? What did they bring to writing and reading by way of their attitudes about literacy? What was the nature of their experiences of school? And what did teachers of teen mothers have to say about their experiences of working with this population? I've answered some of the smaller questions that resided within those larger ones as well.

Along the way I've churned up new questions and made some discoveries. I've uncovered questions about the entrenched middle-class quality of our system of education, about the possibilities of conversations between people from different socioeconomic levels, and about how teachers' deeply ingrained and unconscious middle-class assumptions and values might affect their relationships with working-class students. I've learned that the effects of poverty are far more diffuse, wide ranging, and difficult to pin down than I had realized, affecting family life and personal goals and attitudes toward childbirth and child rearing, and infecting some young women with a hopelessness that may sometimes make their actions confusing to those of us comfortably situated in middle-class lives. I discovered some of the reasons a poor young woman might decide to quit school—reasons that have something to do with the ways schools define intelligence, but also with students' inability to find the right kind of caring in systems where the values privileged are far different from those privileged at home. I've discovered how unprotected from their fellow students' harassment some less well-off students feel.

I've discovered also how important the discourses that surround us are, both at the personal level, influencing how I read and interpreted the words of Casey and Angel, influencing how some teachers treat less well-off female students and how I treated my students all those years ago at the Teen Moms' Program. Discourses are important at the political level as well, influencing the thinking of those who make important educational policy. Who wants to provide help to a teen mother if she's seen as a welfare queen? Who wants to fund a daycare center in a school building if schools are not seen as places that concern themselves with the kind of practical, caretaking work a daycare center would provide? Who wants to help the poor if the poor are seen as having made their own difficulties?

I also learned how social a thing a literate life can be—not like the decontextualized reading and writing valorized by so many standardized tests—and I learned about the importance of the talk around reading and writing—those conversations in which students can test and weigh fact and value, share information, and discover the meanings of their reading and writing, and the meanings of their lives, together. I learned how disorienting it can be for a working-class girl to read a book whose implied reader is a young woman from the middle class.

I also learned about the importance of schools that work against valorizing middle-class students and middle-class ways of living. I've learned about the importance of schools like the Alyssa and Thomas Jefferson Learning Centers, neither of which offered a perfect education, nor a perfect solution to the difficulties working and parenting students have earning an education, but which do provide a partial solution, which is far, far, better than none.

I've heard about the ideas of teachers of teen mothers, who would like to see schools expand to provide more services for their clientele. I've heard from teen mothers who want equitable educations, not educations at schools which treat their pregnancies like a cold to be cured quickly and then brushed aside, or like a contamination (Pillow, 2004, 221) that requires them to be separated from other students. I've heard from students who say that having their children was the best thing they ever did, and who want to be treated with the respect they deserve.

Wanda Pillow quotes Nancy Lesko who asks, "In order to create independent young single mothers, what kinds of programs are necessary?"(quoted in Pillow 2004, 219). She asks what equal might look like in a program for pregnant and mothering teens, and whether anyone even really wants fully independent young single mothers in our society. She positions research about pregnant and mothering teens in schools clearly as "an education gender and race equity issue" (220), suggesting that if we were going to try to provide an equal education for all students, we would have to think about socioeconomic, race, and gender equality in new and imaginative ways.

Summary of General Findings

This study of a small group of teen mothers, and these conversations with a few of the people who have taught them, suggests findings that warrant that attention of teachers and principals, teacher educators, and policy makers. These findings warrant the attention of school workers at both traditional and alternative high schools as well. The general findings I list below fall into three overlapping categories. The first category concerns teen mothers and their literacy learning. The second concerns teen mothers and high school experiences. The third concerns the needs and thoughts of those who teach teen mothers—as most of us will, at some point in our teaching lives.

Literacy and Teen Mothers

The young women with whom I spoke were aware of the stereotypes surrounding teen mothers; though they were not critical of those stereotypes as they were presented in the young-adult novels we read, they didn't necessarily identify with the teen mothers in the novels we read, either. More motivated to graduate from high school than they had ever been, the young women with whom I spoke revealed rich outside-of-school literate lives.

1. The young women with whom I read had some resistance toward seeing themselves as the writers of young-adult fiction depicted them—with good reason, as the writers for the most part presented teen mothers within entrenched and overly simple discourses, as either bad or confused girls, living irresponsible or ineffective lives.

2. The young women with whom I wrote were very aware of the discourses

that surround teenaged motherhood—though they wouldn't have used the language I do!—and were very aware of the ways other people saw them; they were struggling against and within those discourses and toward some kind of dignity as they told and wrote stories of their lives.

3. The young women with whom I read and wrote were more motivated to develop literate lives than they had ever been before. The time shortly after childbirth seems to be a time of increased motivation and force for many young women, as many other researchers have discovered; knowing this, policy makers and administrators could find ways of capitalizing on this motivated period of time to help young mothers who are students learn.

4. Though not always the most proficient readers, these young women tended to have rich outside-of-school literate lives; school workers need to develop ways of capitalizing on such outside-of-school literacies.

Class, Teen Mothers, and School

The working-class young women with whom I spoke revealed surprising reasons for leaving school; they revealed a surprising hunger for knowledge as well. All of the working-class girls had dropped out of school before they became pregnant; in a reverse of the conventional wisdom, it was the birth of their children that caused them to return. All of the young women who continued on in traditional schools revealed some difficulties going to school as pregnant or mothering students.

1. Some working-class students sometimes leave school because they do not feel that the school is a caring environment for them. This sense of being an outsider seems to be promoted primarily by peers; in part this seems to be because of the middle-class values around which traditional schools are structured.

2. Despite the 1975 enactment of Title IX, young women who are pregnant and trying to finish high school are still discriminated against by peers and some teachers and administrators. The traditional high school is not set up well to respect diversity, and as young mothers are living lives outside of conventional norms, unarticulated prejudices and fears cause expressions of discrimination against them.

3. These young mothers are hungry for adults to talk to and hungry for learning as well; schools and administrators and policy makers need to find ways to feed that hunger.

4. The working-class young mothers with whom I spoke had not left school because they became pregnant; rather they came back to school because

they were pregnant or had children. Having children often improved the young mothers' lives in other ways as well.

Teachers of Teen Mothers and School Change

The teachers of teen mothers with whom I spoke saw their students as having particular needs; they wanted the schools in which their students matriculated to change, and described those changes in some detail.

1. The teachers of teen mothers with whom I spoke argued for the value of "full-service" schools, with daycare center, health care center, and other social services located in or near the school building.

2. The main change that teachers of teen mothers wanted was a daycare center housed in the school building. This, they argued, would help the babies receive needed care, help the parents find respite from the never-ending demands of infants, provide the parents with models of nurturing infant care, and perhaps provide models and opportunities for other students to learn about and express care.

Pedagogical and curricular implications

Talking with these young women and their teachers, and reading young-adult novels with them, has given me ideas about kinds of curricula that might help pregnant and mothering teens develop more literate lives. Atwell-Vasey and others describe the importance of the relationship of the body to reading, the body which we so often ignore in traditional teaching. I suggest some ways, inspired by Atwell-Vasey and others, that the pregnant teen's changing body might be seen positively, and as a motivator for literacy learning in the classroom. Next I describe other ways in which reading and writing might be shown to be useful in classrooms where young women want to discuss their changing and challenging lives as new mothers. I also describe the continuing importance of classroom conversations about the affect of media in our lives. Finally, I argue for a political education for pregnant and mothering teens. While many of these curricular innovations would be most easily enacted in what Wanda Pillow (2004) describes as the "single-sex space" of the school or classroom for pregnant and mothering teens (224), many of these ideas about curricula would easily be implemented in traditional schools as well.

Reading and the Body

Adam Phillips (1993) writes that understanding the body is a major job of adolescence:

To the adolescent it is, like the analyst in the transference, the most familiar stranger. In puberty the adolescent develops what can be accurately referred to as transference to his own body; what crystallizes in adolescence, what returns partly as an enactment through risk, are doubts about the mother and the holding environment of infancy. These doubts are transferred onto the body, turned against it, as it begins to represent a new kind of internal environment, a more solitary one. That is to say, the adolescent begins to realize that the original mother is his body.

It is not that the adolescent is attempting to "own his body"—that absurd commodity of ego-psychology—as part of separation from his mother, nor is he simply taking over her care giving aspects. He is testing the representations of the body acquired through early experience. Is it a safe house? Is it reliable? Does it have other allegiances? What does it promise, and what does it refuse? (pp. 31–32)

This testing of the body, this connecting of the experience of the body to "the holding environment of infancy," could be particularly problematic for young women who, like Casey and Angel, have had abusive or intrusive parents or partners in the past. Sue Turnbull (1999) is wise to remind us that the question of "what to do with personal knowledge in the classroom" is complicated, and that all of us need to be tactful and cautious when imposing our ideologies on our students, who may be "caught between desire and duty" (103) as the young women Astrid and Leah, whom Turnbull defends in her article are, or rebellious, claustrophobic and confused, as Casey describes herself being in the classroom.

But part of the testing of the body that Phillips refers to above, and part of the body's promise, was surely, for the young women with whom I spoke, a testing through and a promise of sex. Some conversation about that testing and that promise should be made available in safe spaces, whether in all-girl after-school book groups similar to the one I conducted; in one-on-one conversations, or in small groups in traditional co-ed classrooms. Most female students—even students who already have children—need to have opened up for them that "discourse of desire" that Michelle Fine (1988) describes as being absent from traditional school sex education classes. In traditional schools, such a discourse might be made available through the reading of fiction about pregnant and mothering teens in parenting, health, or English classes, in connection with visits by teen mothers, school nurses, or social workers. Reading fiction about pregnant and mothering teens might open up conversations about the problems and pleasures of female desire; such conversations could help young women think out what they want from the men in their lives and how they might negotiate for what they want. But there are other ways of making the body, and not necessarily the sexual body, a subject in the classroom as well.

According to Wendy Atwell-Vasey (1998), the body is with us whenever we read; she says we read as bodies, we "project our bodies into the time and space of the novel and we feel it or live it from there" (75). Atwell-Vasey also claims that "thought is inextricably bound to the body and the body inextricably bound to thought" (70). The body and its importance to the adolescent and to reading has most often been left out of the classroom. The teenaged mother Winnie spoke of how much more comfortable teachers seemed to be with her after her baby was born, because they didn't have to see evidence of her mothering self, her swollen body, every day in the classroom; Wanda Pillow (2004) writes of pregnant young women trying to fit into desks not made with their bodies in mind (xxi). Situations like these could, particularly in an all-girl classroom, be brought up and interrogated in discussions: What messages do teen mothers feel are being sent to them by these absences and attempts at erasure?

As teen mothers and pregnant teens begin to develop new relationships with their bodies—as they learn who they are as pregnant (Luttrell 2003, 116), as they experience the weight gain, the taking of urine samples, the swollen breasts, the internal experiences of the baby; as they learn about their own "inside stories" (67) of pregnancy, and experience what Raphel-Leff describes as the "strange union of two bodies, one inside the other" (quoted in Luttrell 2003, 67), their relationships to their bodies as readers may change. As the adolescent, and particularly the adolescent mother, is working to understand her body as a safe (or not-so-safe) house, how can we help the adolescent read in new ways? How can we help her work with her body in the classroom and not ignore it? Atwell-Vasey asks how the teacher can "employ body-knowers rather than knowers for whom the body is irrelevant or in the way" (70).

Both Luttrell and Atwell-Vasey answer the question of how to bring the body back into the classroom by suggesting a more prominent place for drama: ". . . since the body makes thought, speech, reading, and writing possible, the use of gesture and theatre ought to be an integral and central dimension of classroom literary practice" (Atwell-Vasey 1998, 69). Wendy Luttrell, in working with pregnant teens in the PPT program, encouraged students to perform and videotape skits in which they wrote about their experiences as pregnant teens. These young women's self-representations, their enactments as storytellers (Luttrell 2003, 114) provided the researcher with insights into the young women's identity-making while also providing the young women with new ways to construct the narratives of their lives (114). The girls wrote and acted out skits in which they defended their moral selves to inconsiderate nurses, or in which they told their mothers they were pregnant (127). In these stories, Luttrell suggests, the girls were both

> wrestling with multiple positions—as victims of stereotype and mistreatment, as vulnerable to men's deceit, as daughters who fear disappointment and loss, and as decision makers who have not chosen the conditions under which they take action (16).

More opportunity for this kind of self-presentation should be made available to pregnant and mothering teens in the classroom.

Other kinds of conversations about the body might be invited by using other kinds of technology: In creating "photo stories" or "identity portraits" (Buckingham & Sefton-Green, 1994, 85), students might explore not only the codes and conventions of different forms of narration (88), not only the connection between the form of the story they create and its meaning (91), but also experience an objectification of themselves, in particular of their bodies, that might engage interesting questions about where the self resides—in the body?—and "how we inscribe the 'self' into different forms of writing and of how we use writing to create different forms of ourselves" (98).

A conversation about mothering and the body of the mother might be made available in all-women classes as well. The young women with whom I spoke had, for the most part, little awareness of and language for conversations around feminist thought ("Is that like—women's lib—like—equal pay?" Angel asked me, and Gabriel described how women, because they menstruate, could not make good soldiers), but movement toward discussions about the valuing of the girl child and the female body of the mother might be possible in a class full of young women like Angel and Gabriel, young women who are mothers or anticipating motherhood.

Other Conversations about Reading in School

In classes where most of the students are not pregnant or mothering, young-adult novels about teen mothers could be used to provide a springboard for discussion of gender expectations and stereotypical representations of teen mothers and their boyfriends. In traditional classrooms conversations about the fact that most of these books were written by women might be fruitful; students might, as Seelinger Trites (2000) suggests, attempt feminist readings of some of these novels, discussing ways in which these novels might be about "female education, female identity formation, female voice, and female choice" (151). Students might begin to talk about whether they believe that women's morality and ideas about relationships are the same or different from those of men. Boys in a co-ed classroom might be interested in defending themselves against the often flat and negative depictions of boyfriends in young-adult novels about teen pregnancy.

Teachers might also begin after-school book clubs, like the one I created, expressly for pregnant and mothering students. In such a book club, through reading some of the texts described here, a teacher might, as Deirdre Kelly suggests, open up a conversation about "the meanings of being a mother, a student, a worker, and a citizen in today's society. Students could compare the competing images of the good mother . . . and discuss who benefits and who is marginalized by such images" (147). Such a conversation could start, perhaps, with the images of the mothers of the teens in the novels I read here—Hannah's troubled mother, Verna LaVaughn's critical mother, and Imani's preoccupied mother—and move on to the kinds of mothers the teens seem to be themselves. As part of this conversation students could look at the images of school in these novels, ask whether school is idealized in each novel or not; they could ask why mothers are still willing to send their children off to an institution such as school (Grumet quoted in Pitt 2006, 101).

Similarly, a conversation about different kinds of knowledge—the difference, as Luttrell (1997) phrases it, between "school-smarts"—the kind of book learning valorized in our schools—and "mother-wisdom"—a form of common sense, a genre of knowledge that has to do with insight and intuition as well as experience gained from watching mothers and grandmothers work with children (31)—might become a rich one. Likewise, in classroom conversations students might compare body-knowledge and mind-knowledge, representational knowledge as opposed to experiential knowledge, as well as other kinds of intelligences.

Media, Literacy Learning, and Teen Mothers

> As we know, a woman's body is endlessly objectified in all the visual media.
>
> —Benjamin 1988, 124.

All students must contend with and learn to read the many media productions around them. I suggest that this learning might be particularly important for young women who are single mothers. Electronic media and popular culture texts may provide a rich language for teen mothers to enjoy, manipulate, and make meaning from, a language richer than any provided by other texts easily available to them. Brenda spoke of how difficult it was for her to get to the library after work, but soap operas were—right there! David Buckingham (2003) reinforces this sense that media texts are readily available to working-poor students when he describes the easy access his research subjects had to all kinds of electronic media (19). Buckingham's description of the availability of media reinforces Robert Yagelski's (2000) suggestion that teenaged readers are changing as the world we live in is changing:

> . . .Technologies now provide instant access to information and events that are themselves a function of those technologies. For instance, in a bizarre kind of irony that seems to prove French philosopher Jean Baudrillard's (1983) arguments about appearance and reality, modern political conventions, so long a crucial part of the election process in American society, are now shaped by television and print media in astounding technological efforts to use those same media to shape public opinion: Television represents television representing reality. It all becomes, to use Baudrillard's term, simulacra. (13)

When Angel describes learning about labor on "the pregnancy channel," instead of from a doctor, midwife, or mother, when she describes her boyfriend's mother videotaping the birth of her son ("but from the side, I didn't want any crotch shots"), when, with Casey and Brenda, she compares her real-life experiences to the experiences of the characters in *CSI* or *Crossing Jordan*, she is providing opportunities a teacher might take up. Teachers might start, simply, as Buckingham does, with a survey of the devices that are in their students' homes, then talk with these students about how in our present society people watch themselves watching themselves, how we create media images of ourselves for the people we will be in the future to watch, and what this might do to our sense of reality.

Certainly we must educate students about how media in our capitalist culture shapes our desires. Yagelski (2000) writes that teenagers have watched "an endless stream of slightly different versions of the same text, the same continuous advertisement for a consumer culture in which agency is defined as the ability to choose which products to buy," and he asks a good question about those experiences, which is, "How does one 'read' these texts, which suggest that the only real power a student . . . has is her purchasing power?" (6). Students need to be helped to answer questions like these, but they need more than this. Media education has gone beyond the attempts to inoculate students against popular culture's dangerous ideologies, whether the attempts come from the right or the left (Buckingham 2003, 125; Tobin 2000, 3); many teachers realize that students are more sophisticated consumers of media images than their teachers are.

One avenue for educating students or helping students educate themselves about media literacy is to help students become producers as well as consumers of media culture. Researchers have argued about the educative value of media production, what Buckingham and Sefton-Green (1994) call "practical" work (184). Is "practical work" merely imitative of popular culture, repeating all its ideologies, or is it creative? To what degree is such work personal, to what degree social (186)? In students' mimicking of popular media forms, is there also critique (185)? Buckingham writes that students should imitate media they are invested in, which suggests that teen mothers might look at and perhaps imitate, in any production work, popular work they know and think about in their everyday lives: for the Angel and Casey, perhaps, parenting magazines or books about child rearing, the shows on the "pregnancy channel," videos watched at the Young Parents' Network meetings. Buckingham and Sefton-Green (1994) point out that students may work in a parodic mode without being fully aware of or, perhaps, able to articulate exactly what it is that they are ridiculing (199). Somewhere in between the play of such work and the reflection on it lies its educative value (199).

Other researchers, like Wendy Luttrell (2003), have described the value of schoolwork that involves play "not in the consumerist sense but . . . in the imaginative, symbol-formation sense" (179) as well as schoolwork that involves pleasure, intuition, art-making and sharing (180). Luttrell writes of how this kind of playful work can help resolve different kinds of binaries—between work and play, between adult and adolescents, between voice and silence. For students for whom traditional schooling has not worked well, such kinds of production work may be of value, not because it is hands-on and therefore presumed to be less rigorous, but because it might tap into kinds of intelligence that are less well served by more print-dependent kinds of learning.

Sue Turnbull (1999) rightly warns readers about the difficulty, for some students, of negotiating the "different sets of expectations" set up by teachers and by parents, particularly, perhaps, students from cultures other than those of the white middle class (100). Turnbull reminds teachers that taste is personal, and that certain discourses that students get great pleasure from—like the discourse of romance—may be disapproved of by teachers. As Alvermann et al. (1999) remind us, teachers and students need to be cognizant that audiences are complicated: Experiences that give one person in the audience pleasure will not necessarily be pleasurable to another person in the audience (33). If teen mothers explore themselves as audiences for popular culture texts, and if by doing so they do research "on their own behalf" (Buckingham 2003, 110) and begin to define themselves and their tastes as both constructed by larger social forces and as individual and personal statements (117), they might begin to trouble the notion of the passive audience, and the passive girl.

In English classes for teen mothers, as in English classes for all students, as Bruce Pirie (1997) writes, "our mandate ought to be the study of textuality: how the network of representations work and how we work it" (23). We need to help young women read the many (media) texts that are using them and that are being used by them; we need to help them see how the meaning of a story changes according to who is telling that story, and why (32).

Perhaps this consideration of media in teens' lives might change the more traditional texts they read as well. In the conservative young-adult texts I read with Casey and Angel there was very little consideration of the affect of media on either the young mothers who are characters in those novels or on the adolescents who will read those novels. Only *Imani All Mine*—of all of the young-adult novels mentioned in this book—made any mention of media images and how they affect its characters, and, again, *Imani All Mine* is a book not written explicitly for teenagers. Writers of young-adult-novels have begun to address issues of media and electronic technology (*Feed* by M.T. Anderson has interesting things to say about adolescents' wired life, for example; *Monster* by Walter Dean Myers uses its main character's videography skills to tell the story) but none of the texts written explicitly about teen mothers that I have read address this new complexity that the multiplicity of media images brings. So I argue here also for more complex representations of the world teen mothers live in—the media-saturated world—in the young-adult texts written about pregnant and mothering teens.

Political Conversations and Literacy Learning

Following Yagelski (2000), I argue also for the political education of teen mothers. Pregnant and mothering teens need to be provided with political skills and the opportunity to use them; pregnant and mothering teens need literacy skills that will help them read about the welfare reform laws that affect their lives, about the transferring of funds from an alternative school that has served them well, about the closing of a daycare center near their school. They need to be provided, by their teachers and their schools, with the sense of confidence that would allow them to act on such reading and encourage them to serve their communities in ways more direct and pertinent to their own needs than just joining in on teen parent panels or teaching in a daycare center. Like the teens at the Youth Eager for Truth school in Utah and at other alternative schools around the country, teen mothers need to be provided opportunities to argue for the continuance of the schools that serve them, to meet with local lawmakers and social workers, to write letters to the editor and circulate petitions, and to argue for structures that will help them live easier, more dignified lives.

School Structures, School Change, and Nontraditional Students

Conversations with teachers of teen mothers and other nontraditional students have suggested the need not only for continuing and fuller funding of alternative schools, like the Thomas Jefferson and Alyssa Learning Centers and the Teen Moms' Program, which service students who are often less well off, working, or mothering; but also changes to traditional schools that are deep and far-reaching. If all schools could be made more "full service," combining "the school with the settlement house," and if we could loosen the hold of the Carnegie unit, even traditional schools would move toward becoming more equitable places for married, pregnant, and mothering teens, and for other nontraditional students as well.

Working-Class Students, Girls, and Sports

Lisa Dodson (1998) writes that poor girls are needed to help their families at home, so that they are often unable to participate in after-school sports clubs, arts clubs, and other programs that might widen their world. She writes that poor girls need to be granted a "family work release" (215) in order to be involved in these activities that might provide them with new visions of themselves as well as contacts with adults who have different skills. Similarly, Wanda Pillow (2004, 224) describes how middle-class women are most often the students who engage in sports teams in school. (I think of Brenda, who joined a sports club but dropped out after she was harassed because of her less-than-hip clothes, her diction; I think of Winnie, who was an award-winning gymnast.) Both Dodson and Pillow suggest that if they could participate in after-school sports clubs, or indeed other clubs, poor young women might develop different relationships to their bodies, and different images of themselves that would not make early childbirth look like the only way to prove their competence and adulthood. Ensuring that all facilities—including after-school facilities like sports teams—were available to all students could be seen as another part of becoming a school that is "full service."

Success in School, Time, and Social Capital

We must also work toward new ways of defining success in school. Presently, it seems, we define success largely in terms of time. If students graduate from high school in four years, they are considered successes. But don't we all want students who are, as Beth describes the students at Thomas Jefferson, "goal-oriented and focused?" If we truly believe in the good of the concept of lifelong education, who provides a better image of the successful student than these focused, goal-oriented students who "keep coming back" so that they can finish their degrees, however many years that takes?

More simply, young mothers and other nontraditional students need to be helped, through school-based service-learning, or mentoring programs, to develop social capital—that series of social networks that creates connections that can help people meet others who can help them, in small and large ways, and that can help us all feel safe and protected in our worlds (Noguera 2003, 34; Schultz 2001, 604). I was continually struck by the isolation of the young women with whom I worked. Casey, Angel, and Brenda had children and mothers, boyfriends or husbands, but often times these people were not available to help them through the complicated and new experiences of birthing and raising a baby. The burdens of poverty fell hard upon the relatives of some of these young women, and the amount of time and effort it took relatives to make it through a regular day meant that time for important conversations was often just not there. The support these relatives did provide was complicated—whether by the youth, arrogance, and selfishness of a boyfriend, the preoccupation of a soon-to-be-laid off bartender mother, or the different age of a husband. Schools could provide multiple ways for pregnant and mothering students—whether they are poor or middle class—find adults who might show them new ways of living in the world, and provide new connections.

School workers need to be encouraged to think about developing a definition of independence for young mothers that moves beyond simple employment (Lesko, quoted in Pillow 2004); school workers need to be encouraged to imagine the kinds of classes, curricula, and overall programs that teen mothers might need in order to become single mothers with control over their lives (Pillow 2004, 219). We must encourage school administrators, as Katherine Schultz writes, to look at how their schools "limit the possibilities they offer to female students" (2001, 604), and we must move beyond just a reduction of limitations toward new as-yet-unthought-of structures and possibilities as well. We must show educators and policy makers the ineffectuality of their tendency to "carve away the complexities" (Schultz 2001, 604) when talking and writing about the education of teen mothers.

If it's true that "a major goal in life—perhaps the major goal in life—is to discover or compose the right story for one's own life" (McAdams 1989, 28), then we need schools and teachers who can help nontraditional students think critically about how to find those right stories in a country that so often doesn't allow young women to define their own sexuality, that doesn't provide working-poor students much economic hope, or value, in traditional schools at least, experiential knowledge. We need schools like the Thomas Jefferson and Alyssa Learning Centers—and schools better than those—where teachers help young mothers and other nontraditional students critique and question their world, collect the knowledge they desire, and begin to learn how to think themselves toward freedom.

Alfreda, whom I met early on at the Thomas Jefferson Learning Center, assured me that time spent with her would be time well spent. "You want to listen to me, oh yes you do," she said, "because I've got stories to tell. I'm eighteen, I have four kids, I'm trying to finish school, and I've got a lot of stories." We would be wise to listen to the stories these young women tell.

Where Are They Now?

What became of Angel and Casey, Gabriel and Brenda? What choices did Beth Manning and Melinda Vane make, and what happened to the Alyssa and Thomas Jefferson Learning Centers? Several years after I conducted the research this book describes I searched out these women, some of whom I was still in touch with daily, and some of whom I had not heard from since my research was finished.

I found both Angel and Casey—you won't be surprised—on Facebook. Angel sounds quite happy; she's still together with, though not yet married to, her soul mate Jason. Jason and Angel have four children—three shining little golden-haired girls as well as Ben, who is in second grade: two of his baby teeth just fell out. Angel loves her kids, her immediate and extended family, and getting together with her friends to have a good time. She's been working on learning to cook big and really nutritious meals for her family. She hasn't finished high school yet, and she's looking for a job.

Casey looks happy in her Facebook photo; graceful and thoughtful and tall, she's sitting with her son Russ on a checkered blanket out in a neighborhood park. She tells me that she graduated with her GED in 2006, and that she's still happily married to Sam, who now works for the power company. Casey writes that her son is in first grade and "at the top of his class," and that she stays at home to care for him and his younger sister full time. Her mother—the mother who cried every night when Casey was living with foster parents—is one of her "top" Facebook friends.

I hear from others that Brenda moved through the courses the local community college set before her with characteristic energy and enthusiasm. For a time after she began at the community college, she came by the Thomas Jefferson Learning Center in the afternoons. There her former teachers helped her with the writing of papers, which she knew to be her greatest weakness; later, Brenda found tutoring help at the composition department at the community college. She has graduated now—her dream fulfilled—and works as a licensed practical nurse in the area.

It took me a while to find Melinda, the administrator who had worked in the Career Room of the Alyssa Learning Center. I learned, first, that the Alyssa Learning Center had been shut down when the Republican state senate reduced its funding; concerns that the school was not meeting the many regulations required by *No Child Left Behind* may have played some part in the school's closing. Through a mutual friend, I learned that Melinda had been upset by the closing of the center; she worried about the students the program used to serve. But she had been earning credits toward her master's degree in counseling in the evenings, and found work as a guidance counselor at one of the wealthier high schools in Alyssa. She's very happy—"ecstatic!" is how our mutual friend put it—in her new position.

Beth quit work at the Thomas Jefferson Learning Center after a student threatened her late one night. She was the only adult in the building, and though she had set up a system where she could easily call the police to come and help her should any student become violent, that system failed. Despite conversations with the director of the high school program about ways in which they might make the center a safer place for teachers and administrators to work, her supervisors decided not to put money into making these changes. With some regret, Beth chose to move to a job in another area of education. Some years later the funding for serving high school students through the Thomas Jefferson Learning Center was greatly reduced; at the Center now fewer students earn their GEDs, and they earn them through online courses.

Many of the young women I worked with had transient lives: cell phone numbers and addresses changed, boyfriends came and went, parents sometimes moved, too. Calling a number and finding that it was no longer in service was a common occurrence. Though the lives of the teachers who worked with these young women were of a far different quality than the lives of the teen mothers, the teachers often lived unsettled lives as well. Teaching students whose lives don't conform to middle-class norms is still not a national priority—despite our new president. With an educational establishment that prioritizes the schooling of middle-class students, alternative schools close down or sputter on under-funded; eventually, some teachers find that, like their students, they need to move on.

Methodology

This book began with the notebooks I filled when I was a young teacher at the school I've called the Teen Moms' Program. Three of the interludes in this book came from those notebooks, as well as from letters I sent to my mother during that year. Clearly, I've shaped the notes to my own interests, making them reflect subjects I've focused on in the researched chapters. Though I've only presented some of my notes, I hope that these interludes, not really qualitative research, not exactly triangulated or backed up with statements from experts, do suggest some of the immediate experiences of a young teacher working in an unusual setting. It's my hope that these brief interludes can provide teachers who are young now with the solace of knowing that we have all made mighty mistakes in our attempts to reach students, perhaps especially, for middle-class teachers, those students who live "out on the borderlands" (Steedman 1986). It's my hope as well that these small notes can help readers learn a bit about what the curriculum was like in the single-sex space where I worked; I hope that these notes can show that one space, at least, included some of that "woman-centered talk, curriculum, and pedagogy" Wanda Pillow (2004, 226) worries is "glaringly" absent from schools for pregnant and mothering teens. These interludes might also suggest some of what a young teacher needs to know when she's working in such a space, and some of all the many things she might learn.

In the methodology section of her strong and beautiful book *Don't Call Us Out of Name*, Lisa Dodson (1998) writes that she disagrees with the traditional argument that researchers must retain positions of neutrality in their investigations. She states that she believes that "neutrality is a false position for anyone, researcher or not." She describes the importance of what she calls "crossing over" which involves spending "considerable time" with the people being researched, and "learning the lessons of engagement" as well. She writes that "when you look into the faces of women raising their children in the outback, you see that neutrality is not recognized as some professional practice. In the face of stigma, irrational regulations, peril to children, and a woman's despair, neutrality is known only as collusive silence" (246).

I hope this book expresses some of the difficulty and importance, for teachers, of such crossing over. I hope this book counters some of the simplistic presentations of the working poor in teacher education materials today. I describe my own reactions to the young women I got to know not to focus on myself in particular but as a way to explore the complexity of the experience of teaching today, when society's definition of what schools should do and what teachers should be has become increasingly narrow.

Like most researchers, in order to protect privacy, I changed the names of every person written about in this book, and often other distinguishing details about their lives. Though I asked Brenda, Casey, Gabriel, Angel, Beth, and Melinda to choose the names that they are called by in this text, I made up the names of others, and of the girls and the teachers I knew at the Teen Moms' Program. I am grateful to all of them for their time and their willingness to share their stories with me.

I have been reading and thinking about pregnant, married, and mothering teens for many years. The fact that my perspective on teen mothers changed from the time I was a teacher of teen mothers to the time when I was a mother myself, and a researcher on the subject, perhaps suggests that we need more mothers in places of educational power.

Data Sources and Collection

I conducted this research over several years and wrote it up as a series of separate studies. In the fall and winter of 2002 and the spring of 2003 I spent thirty hours interviewing teachers of teen mothers, asking them about their experiences working with teen mothers in the schools, what they would like to see changed in both the education of the young women they knew and in the structure of the schools they worked in, as well as what they thought the ideal school for teen parents might be. I conducted semi-structured interviews with Nathan Smith, Beth Manning, Melinda Vane, Jenny Moore, Juliette Baldwin, and Nettie Hacker, an administrator at the Thomas Jefferson Learning Center. In many different venues I heard the stories of Letitia Moss, and through Letitia I found Carol Jones, an English teacher in the GOALS program in Ohio; Carol and I talked primarily about activities she conducted and texts she used when she taught English to pregnant and mothering teens.

I also spoke with teen mothers themselves. In the winter of 2003 and the spring of 2004 I conducted multiple four-hour-long interviews with two older women, Jennifer Bowles and Beth Manning, who described their experiences as teen mothers many years ago; I also spoke extensively, in the winter of 2002, with Winnie Jones, who was navigating the halls of a traditional high school.

The heart of this research was conducted, though, with Casey Howard, Angel Brown, Brenda Parker, and Gabriel Banks at the Thomas Jefferson Learning Center and the Alyssa Learning Center. It is these women I spent most time with—over fifty hours, during the spring and summer semesters of 2003 and beyond—both in the book club, listening to their reactions, in casual, weekly conversations, and in semi-structured interviews. Because I was much older than these women I wielded a certain power; I tried not to present myself as a teacher, I tried to undercut my own authority in our conversations; still the differences in age and status surely influenced the responses I received from Casey, Angel, Brenda, and Gabriel.

Analysis

From these different studies I collected data sources which included audio taped book club discussions, interviews with students, teachers, counselors, and administrators, field notes taken throughout the semesters, students' written responses to literature, students' written essays, and some administrative records. I analyzed these data sources in a variety of ways. As I read and reread my typed transcripts, as I studied my pages of field notes, I identified recurring patterns in the data, as well as similar comments made by more than two people. I noticed, for example, how often the young women described school as a way to climb up the socioeconomic ladder, as well as how often the young women's values, habits, and ways of speaking seemed foreign to me. Under the category of "language" I placed comments the women made about learning how to talk "right" in school; under the category of "SES in school," I placed stories about unfair treatment at the hands of teachers, administrators, and other students. Under the category of "money" I placed comments about buying shoes for children, affording college, and using food stamps. I created a sometimes-overlapping category called "upward mobility" because three of the women spoke frequently about how they hoped to improve their financial situations. I searched for disconfirming evidence as well, learning about the socioeconomic status of the middle-class women I spoke to.

I conducted narrative analyses on the life stories and reading histories the teenage mothers shared with me. I asked the young women about their childhoods, their earliest memories of reading and writing, their first experiences in school, their relationships with their parents and with any particular teachers. I asked the young women what their current home lives were like and what their most important relationships were. I asked what they would tell teen mothers and teachers of teen mothers if they could, and what they thought the best kind of schooling would have been for them. I asked them to tell me the stories of their lives.

Following Stan Wortham's (2001) suggestions in *Narratives in Action*, I tried to determine the different kinds of voices in which the young mothers were speaking, and the various societal conversations into which they were directing their stories. I looked for metaphors, repetitions, nicknames, Freudian slips, and for words that seemed to come from a different voice in the young women's talk as I read and reread transcripts of our conversations. Using the work of Wortham and Ochs and Capps, I thought about the ways in which the students were performing for me, and what their different ways of presenting themselves to me at each of our meetings might mean.

Lisa Dodson (1998) writes that "life-history interviews are particularly complicated ethically and personally. They are deeply revealing, and when you listen to the lives of poor women in America, the revelations often call for a response" (249). I've written in earlier pages about the unnerving and enervating experience of feeling that expectation, that yearning for a response. I tried to steer the young women I spoke with toward people and institutions that might help them, and I tried to encourage the women I spoke to do the same for each other. It is true though that I left some of the women I spoke with obviously still in need of other resources.

In some ways this book is a series of recorded conversations. The national conversations about education are dispiriting right now; conversations about the poor seem nonexistent. That makes it all the more important that people from different socioeconomic classes get together in the back of classrooms, in coffeeshops, and libraries and conference rooms to talk about education, and to hear from the young people affected. The conversations in this book, I hope, are examples of some of these kinds of conversations, conversations between poor young mothers and an older mother who is safely a part of the middle class; between tough and thoughtful women and men who are teaching in alternative schools now; between social workers and teachers, and between older women troubled about the ways we are educating young women, and the ways we are treating poor people, our people.

The most important of these conversations, for me, have been with the woman I've called Beth Manning. Her voice is the one most often heard, besides mine, in these pages. She led me into the world of the Thomas Jefferson Learning Center and told me her stories. She described her experiences as a young, single mother, going on and off welfare, working different jobs, building her career and raising her son alone, with determination and joy. She also graciously read this manuscript, corrected my mistakes, and troubled some of my assumptions. She and I have been talking about schools, sex, literacy, justice, and the education of girls and women for over a decade now. I look forward to continuing those conversations for a long time to come.

References

Alvermann, D., Moon, J., & Hagood, M. (1999). *Popular culture in the classroom: Teaching and researching critical media literacy.* Newark and Chicago: The International Reading Association and the National Reading Conference.

Atwell-Vasey, W. (1998). *Nourishing words: Bridging private reading and public teaching.* Albany, New York: SUNY Press.

Baudrillard, J. (1983). *Simulations.* New York: Semiotexte.

Benjamin, J. (1988). *The bonds of love: Psychoanalysis, feminism, and the problem of domination.* New York: Pantheon.

Blackford, H. (2004). *Out of this world: Why literature matters to girls.* New York: Teachers College Press.

Boler, M. (1999). *Feeling power: Emotions and education.* London: Routledge.

Brandt, D. (2001). *Literacy in American lives.* New York: Cambridge University Press.

Brantlinger, E. (2003). *Dividing classes: How the middle class negotiates and rationalizes school advantage.* London: Taylor & Francis.

Britzman, D. (2006). Sigmund Freud, Melanie Klein, and Little Oedipus: On the pleasures and disappointments of sexual enlightenment. In G. Boldt & P. Salvio (Eds.), *Love's return: Psychoanalytic essays on childhood, teaching, and learning* (pp 165–184). New York: Routledge.

Buckingham, D. (2003). *Media education: Literacy, learning and contemporary culture.* Cambridge, UK: Polity.

Buckingham, D., & Sefton-Green, J. (1994). *Cultural studies goes to school: Reading and teaching popular media.* London: Taylor & Francis.

Bunting, E. (2000). *Doll baby.* New York: Clarion.

Bruner, J. (2003). *Making stories: Law, literature, life.* New York: Farrar, Straus & Giroux.

Burke, J. (2000). *Reading reminders: Tools, tips, and techniques.* Portsmouth, NH: Boynton/Cook.

Cherland, M. R. (1994). *Private practices: Girls reading fiction and constructing identity.* London: Taylor & Francis.

Coffel, C. M. (2002). Strong portraits and stereotypes: Images of pregnant and mothering teens in YA fiction. *The ALAN Review* 30, (1), 15–21.

Coffel, C. M. (2009). "I connected so well with it": A teen mother talks about reading. *The International Journal of Qualitative Studies in Education.* 1–6.

Dimen, M. (1994). "Money, love, and hate: Contradiction and paradox in psychoanalysis." *Psychoanalytical Dialogues,* 4, 69–100.

Dodson, L. (1998). *Don't call us out of name: The untold lives of women and girls in poor America.* Boston: Beacon.

Dryfoos, J. (1994). *Full service schools: A revolution in health and social services for children, youth, and families.* San Francisco: Jossey-Bass.

Edin, K., & Kefelas, M. (2005). *Promises I can keep: Why poor women put motherhood before marriage.* Berkeley: University of California Press.

Ellsworth, E. (1997). *Teaching positions: Difference, pedagogy, and the power of address.* New York: Teachers College Press.

Finders, M. (1997). *Just girls: Hidden literacies and life in junior high.* New York: Teachers College Press.

Fine, M. (1988). Schooling, sexuality, and adolescent females: The missing discourse of desire. In M. Fine & L. Weis (Eds.), *Beyond silenced voices: Class, race, and gender in U. S. schools* (pp. 75–99). Albany, NY: SUNY Press.

Hargreaves, A. (1996). *Schooling for change: Reinventing education for early adolescents.* New York: Routledge.

Hargreaves, A. (1997). *Rethinking educational change with heart and mind.* New York: Association for Curriculum and Development.

Hays, S. (2003). *Flat broke with children: Women in the age of welfare reform.* Oxford, UK: Oxford University Press.

Heilbrun, C. (1988). *Writing a woman's life* (pp. 66–82). New York: Ballantine.

Hicks, D. (2002). *Reading lives: Working-class children and literacy learning.* New York: Teachers College Press.

Holland, D., Lachicotte, Jr., W., Skinner, D., & Cain, C. (1998). *Identity and agency in cultural worlds.* Cambridge, MA: Harvard University Press.

Horsman, J. (2000). *Too scared to learn: Women, violence, and education.* Mahwah, NJ: Lawrence Erlbaum.

Keizer, G. (1988). *No place but here: A teacher's vocation in a rural community.* Hanover and London: University Press of New England.

Keizer, G. (2004). *Help: The original human dilemma.* New York: HarperCollins.

Kelly, D. (2000). *Pregnant with meaning: Teen mothers and the politics of inclusive schooling.* New York: Peter Lang.

Lazarre, J. (1980). *On loving men.* New York: Dial Press.

Lesko, N. (1998). Before their time: Social-age, sexuality, and school-aged mothers. In S. Books (Ed.), *Invisible children in the society and its schools* (pp. 121–135). Mahwah, NJ: Lawrence Erlbaum.

Lesko, N. (2001) *Act your age! A cultural construction of adolescence.* London: RoutledgeFalmer.

Luker, K. (1996). *Dubious conceptions: The politics of teenage pregnancy.* Cambridge, MA, and London: Harvard University Press.

Luttrell, W. (1997). *School-smart and mother-wise: Working-class women's identity and schooling.* New York: Routledge.

Luttrell, W. (2003). *Pregnant bodies, fertile minds: Gender, race, and the schooling of pregnant teens.* New York: Routledge.

Luttrell, W., & C. Parker (2001). High school students' literacy practices and identities and the figured world of school. *Journal of Research in Reading*, 24 (3), 235–247.

Lycke, K. (2010). Reading and writing teenage motherhood: Changing literacy practices and developing identities. In L. MacGillivray (Ed.), *Literacy in times of crisis: Practices and perspectives.* New York: Routledge.

McAdams, D. P. 1989. *Intimacy: The need to be close.* New York: Doubleday.

Miller, A. H. (2002a). Reading thoughts: Victorian perfectionism and the display of thinking. *Studies in the Literary Imagination*, 35, 79–88.

Miller, A. H. (2002b). Perfectly helpless. *Modern Language Quarterly*, 63, 65–88.

Musick, Judith (1993). *Young, poor, and pregnant: The psychology of teenage motherhood.* New Haven, CT: Yale University Press.

Newkirk, T. (1992). The narrative roots of the case study. In G. Kirsch & P. Sullivan (Eds.), *Methods and Methodology in Composition Research* (pp. 130–152). Carbondale, IL: Southern Illinois University Press.

Newkirk, T. (1997). *The performance of self in student writing.* Portsmouth, NH: Boynton/Cook.

Noddings, N. (1992). *The challenge to care in schools.* New York: Teachers College Press.

Noguera, Pedro. (2003). *City schools and the American dream: Reclaiming the promise of public education.* New York: Teachers College Press.

Nussbaum, M. (2001). *Upheavals of thought.* Cambridge, UK: Cambridge University Press.

Ochs, E., & Capps, L. (2001). *Living narrative: Creating lives in everyday storytelling.* Cambridge, MA: Harvard University Press.

Pelzer, D. (1995). *A child called "It": One child's courage to survive*. Deerfield Beach, FL: Health Communications.

Phillips, A. (1993). *On kissing, tickling, and being bored: Psychoanalytic essays on the unexamined life*. Cambridge, MA: Harvard University Press.

Pillow, W. (2000). Exposed methodology: The body as a deconstructive practice. In E. A. St. Pierre & W. S. Pillow (Eds.), *Working the ruins: Feminist poststructural theory and methods in education* (pp. 199–219). New York: Routledge.

Pillow, W. (2004). *Unfit subjects: Educational policy and the teen mother*. New York: Routledge.

Pirie, B. (1997). *Reshaping high school English*. Urbana, IL: National Council of Teachers of English.

Pitt, A. (2006). Mother love's education. In G. Boldt & P. Salvio (Eds.), *Love's return: Psychoanalytic essays on childhood, teaching, and learning* (pp. 87–104). New York: Routledge.

Plummer, L. (2000). *A dance for three*. New York: Delacorte.

Porter, C. (1999). *Imani all mine*. Boston: Houghton Mifflin.

Radway, J. A. (1984). *Reading the romance: Women, patriarchy, and popular culture*. Chapel Hill, NC: The University of North Carolina Press.

Ruddick, S. (1989). *Maternal thinking: Towards a politics of peace*. Boston: Beacon.

Ruhlman, M. (1996). *Boys themselves: A return to single-sex education*. New York: Henry Holt.

Schultz, K. (2001, August). Constructing failure, narrating success: Rethinking the "problem" of teen pregnancy. *Teachers College Record, 103,* 582–607.

St. Pierre, E. A. (2000). Poststructural feminism in education: An overview. *International Journal of Qualitative Studies in Education, 13*(5), 477–515.

Trites, R. S. (1997). *Waking sleeping beauty: Feminist voices in children's novels*. Iowa City, IA: University of Iowa Press.

Trites, R. S. (2000). *Disturbing the universe: Power and repression in adolescent literature.* Iowa City, IA: University of Iowa Press.

Tronto, J. (1994). *Moral boundaries; A political argument for an ethic of care.* New York: Routledge.

Solomon, R. C. (1986). Literacy and the education of the emotions. In S. De Castell, A. Luke, & K. Egan (Eds.), *Literacy, society, and schooling: A reader* (pp. 37–58). Cambridge, UK: Cambridge University Press.

Steedman, C. (1986). *Landscape for a good woman: A portrait of two lives.* London: Virago.

Tobin, J. (2000). *Good guys don't wear hats: Children's talk about the media.* New York: Teachers College Press.

Trelease, J. (2006). *The read-aloud handbook.* New York: Penguin.

Turnbull, S. (1999). Dealing with feeling: Why girl number twenty still doesn't answer. *International Journal of Qualitative Studies in Education*, 6, 88–105.

Tyack, D., & Cuban, L. (1995). *Tinkering toward utopia: A century of public school reform.* Cambridge, MA: Harvard University Press.

Tye, B. (2000). *Hard truths: Uncovering the deep structure of schooling.* New York: Teachers College Press.

Vargos Llosa, M. (2001, May). "Why literature?" *The New Republic.*

Vinz, R. (2000). *Becoming (other)wise: Enhancing critical reading perspectives.* Portland, ME: Calendar Island.

Wells, M. C. (1996). *Literacies lost: When students move from a progressive middle school to a traditional high school.* New York: Teachers College Press.

Wolf, V. E. (1993). *Make lemonade.* New York: Scholastic.

Wortham, S. E. (2001). *Narratives in action: A strategy for research and analysis.* New York: Teachers College Press.

Yagelski, R. P. (2000). *Literacy matters: Writing and reading the social self.* New York: Teacher College Press.

Yagelski, R. P. (2009, October). A thousand writers writing: Seeking change through the radical practice of writing as a way of being. *English Education,* (42), 6–28.

Index

W

Y

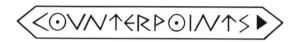

Studies in the Postmodern Theory of Education

General Editor
Shirley R. Steinberg

Counterpoints publishes the most compelling and imaginative books being written in education today. Grounded on the theoretical advances in criticalism, feminism, and postmodernism in the last two decades of the twentieth century, Counterpoints engages the meaning of these innovations in various forms of educational expression. Committed to the proposition that theoretical literature should be accessible to a variety of audiences, the series insists that its authors avoid esoteric and jargonistic languages that transform educational scholarship into an elite discourse for the initiated. Scholarly work matters only to the degree it affects consciousness and practice at multiple sites. Counterpoints' editorial policy is based on these principles and the ability of scholars to break new ground, to open new conversations, to go where educators have never gone before.

For additional information about this series or for the submission of manuscripts, please contact:

Shirley R. Steinberg
c/o Peter Lang Publishing, Inc.
29 Broadway, 18th floor
New York, New York 10006

To order other books in this series, please contact our Customer Service Department:

(800) 770-LANG (within the U.S.)
(212) 647-7706 (outside the U.S.)
(212) 647-7707 FAX

Or browse online by series:
www.peterlang.com